The Comp [illegible] iet For Beginners: A Simple Ketogenic Diet Approach for Rapid Weight loss Plus Keto Diet Meal Plan (2nd Edition)

Part 1

CHAPTER ONE

The History of Ketogenic

During the middle ages, as childhood epilepsy ravaged the strength of juveniles, a burden squared on the shoulders of parents to find a treatment that will stop the suffering to which kids were subjected to. This epilepsy epidemic stood at that time before many like a consuming fire. It must be understood that medicine as at that stage was still in its infancy compared to now where modern medicine can cure almost every form of the disease that tries to plague the lives of men. As the searching for this cure to childhood epilepsy dragged on, the society as at that period started to rely on alternatives to treat their young. Worn out by the scourge of epilepsy that flogged kids to convulsion, people started relying on an ancient model of treatment – fasting as a means of treating seizures. Fasting as a means of holding down raging epilepsy that was fighting furious wars on the body and the brains of kids won an array of successful medallion like a young athlete upon his debut appearance in the sport. This brought hope and joy to the families of many who had sunk deep into the dark tunnel of hopelessness. For them, respite came at last from the insurmountable mountain of convulsion will finally be leveled. The success of this method of treatment gained a higher currency as it was relied upon solely as the means of treating epilepsy in kids in the early 1900's which had hitherto waged savage wars on juveniles at that time.

The Failure of the Early Diet

Though fasting was employed, its efficacy only lasted as long as the fasting continued. Once the fasting is dotted with a pause, epilepsy invaded kids with athletic agility thus rendering fasting only as a yoke that the young of that time must bear to be epilepsy-free. Between the 1900s to the 1920s, modern medicine has to a large extent experienced significant growth that it could be administered to epileptic kids. To what extent were these drugs effective? It was this question that led to the first light of Ketogenic diet to shine forth in 1921. This discovery was shouldered by Doctor Wilder, and it was at the John Hopkins Hospital that this discovery was made.

Trouble Times for the Diet

After a love affair with drugs, the society once again found itself drawn by Ketogenic diet, which in the middle ages could be related to fasting. This diet was majorly on fat, and it restricted carbohydrates intake. However, a wind of change started to blow against the continued survival of this young and formidable diet. As the wind of change blew harder, the rise of Ketogenic diet was crippled by the disfavor that later saluted it. In the U.S, anti-fat campaigns mounted severe pressure on the weak foundation of the

Ketogenic diet. Soon, Ketogenic diet found this pressure too much to bear, and it crumbled to obscurity. These anti-fat campaigns won the day that they received even the U.S government support. The anti-fat campaign's report was later codified in government reports on dietary because of the McGovern Report. Beyond the anti-fat campaigns which had made nonsense of Ketogenic diet as at that time, there was also a breakthrough in the science of medicine in the 30s, 40s, and 50s which seemed to be a viable means of treatment than Ketogenic diet.

A resurrected form of Ketogenic diet with some few modifications called Medium Chain Triglyceride diet found expression, but its usage died as quickly as it came to limelight in 1994.

The True Success Story

As time piled up, the Ketogenic diet was once again able to stage a comeback to the scene with the story of a two-year-old who had had seizures that refused to bow to the control of medications or other forms of treatment including brain surgery. The boy's father hungered by the burning desire to discover more knowledge about the Ketogenic diet started digging up information about the diet. He sought for the information and found it which led to the end of John Hopkins Medical Centre. The boy's seizure was completely controlled as long as he was on a diet. Due to the successful taming of the seizure by the boy's father in administering the diet, he created a foundation which produced many videos, books and sponsored conferences for the training of doctors and diet experts for the implementation of Ketogenic diet. Today, the diet has now become the subject of study in the medical field which is applicable to different types of diseases. Although the Ketogenic diet has gained a lot of acceptance among medical experts, the principal reason for this ton of interest and acceptance is just for one purpose – to find a Ketogenic diet drug.

In the final analysis of this historical discussion, it must be noted that when Ketogenic diet attained the status of media publicity many years ago, so many critics complained that long-term studies on the Ketogenic diet had not been carried out. At present, a sea of studies have been conducted on a diet, and those studies have not established the negative effects of

Ketogenic diet. The Ketogenic diet has been called by different names recently. At present, there are so many researches that have been published pointing to the effectiveness of Ketogenic diet has left so much to be desired.

Explaining Ketogenic Diet

If you have followed me very closely, you would have noticed that we have known relatively what Ketogenic Diet is as a result of the explanation supplied in the introduction. However, I want to give you a definition of what Ketogenic diet means. By definition, Ketogenic diet is a low-carb and high-fat diet in which the amount of carb is lowered, and the amount of fat taken is increased. The primary purpose of the Ketogenic diet is to encourage your body system to stop burning carbs as fuel and burn fat as ketones. This process is achieved by lowering the level of carb intake to 50 grams in a day. But what is ketosis? Ketosis is a metabolic process where the production of ketones by the liver is undertaken. What usually happens when the intake of carbohydrate is lowered is that the body adjusts and shifts into ketosis. A high percentage of cells in the human body utilizes ketones as a source of energy. The usage of ketone bodies by the cells usually occur at a time of long fast or restricted consumption of carbohydrate. Ketones can provide energy for most organs in the body. It is very important to know that glucose is the primary energy for most cells in the body. For the purpose of conserving the use of energy for futuristic use, the body stores excess glucose as glycogen. This glycogen is found in the liver and in the muscle. The glycogen stored in the liver is used to maintain the usual levels of glucose in the blood. In contrast, glycogen that has been stored up are for the purposes of fueling muscle activities. When the intake of carbohydrate restriction is in top gear, protein, as well as fats, can be used as a source of energy. The majority of cells in the body can make use of fatty acids for energy. In a time of shortage or complete lack of carbohydrate, the liver breaks down fat. At such times, ketone bodies can be used by most cells. The production of ketone in excess of what the body requires makes the level of ketones to increase resulting in what is known as ketosis.

What to Know About Ketogenic Diet

When dietary conditions are normal, the human body runs on a combination of the following – carbohydrates, protein, and fat. The moment carbohydrates are eliminated from food that is consumed, the reservoir of carbohydrate in the body are used up. In order to continue working, the body must find an alternative source of energy that it would use as fuel. Among the fuels that the body needs are free fatty acids, which many cells in the body can use. Some cells in the body cannot, however, use Free Fatty Acid. The brain cannot use it. They can make use of ketone bodies. When this free fatty acid is not completely broken down in the liver, ketone bodies are produced. This fatty acid that has not been broken down will serve as a source of fuel for the brain.

Low Carb Diet

- Confusion has arisen that has many people thinking that whenever they are on a diet that is low in carbohydrate, they begin to tell themselves that they are on a Ketogenic diet. This seeming confusion has been compounded by the belief that low carb diet and Ketogenic diet are the same. However, I will explain to you that there is a great difference between these two diets. These differences are as follows:
- The composition of the Diet: This is perhaps is the greatest distinguishable factor between the Ketogenic diet and other diets that are low in carbs. While the Ketogenic diet is majorly a low-carb and high-fat diet, in the case of other forms of diets that are low in carb, it could be low carb and high protein. It is

important to know that your fat level in a low carb diet does not matter since the body runs on carbohydrate as its key fuel source. Conversely, on a Ketogenic diet, about 70 percent of your calories per day are from fat, since fat has now become your primary source of fuel.

- Percentage of Carb Intake: This is another form of the difference between Ketogenic diet and other forms of low carb diet. Many types of research have suggested that eating less than 30% of calories gotten from carbohydrate. That is 50 to about 125 grams of carbs daily. On the other hand, on a Ketogenic diet, the intake of carbohydrate is about 5 to 15% per day and a maximum threshold of 50 grams of carbs.
- The ratio of Weight Loss: It will be important for you to know that the weight lost on the Ketogenic diet is

faster than those experienced in other low carb diets. This is no conjecture or manufacture of facts. In our first difference that was explained above, we have stated that in Ketogenic diet, your intake of carbohydrate is lower than it can be in other forms of low carb diets. While in other diets, your carb can be up to 30%, but in Ketogenic diet, the carb intake can be just 10%. Now looking at the above, who will lose weight faster? Certainly, the person who is on a Ketogenic diet.

- Fuel Source: The source of fuel in the body when a person is on a low carb diet is carbohydrate while in the case of Ketogenic diet, the main source of fuel comes from ketone bodies which are mostly fat.
- Activity Stage: It is important to know that during the time of abundance of carbohydrate source in the

body system, ketone bodies are normally dormant and inactive. As a matter of fact, they are sleeping and do not wake up. However, during the time of shortage of carb and long fasting periods, ketone bodies play a more active role than any form of fuel source. The brain and other cells that make use of predominantly another source of fuel such as carb will switch and begin to use fat.

Similarities

Even though there are many differences between Ketogenic diet and other low carb diets, it is important to know that there are similarities between these two diets. I will make an attempt to explain just a few to you.

- Purpose: No one ever undertakes a low-carb diet or Ketogenic to add more weight. People engage on low carb diet to lose more weight. This is the similarity between Ketogenic diet and low carb diet which is weight loss as their main goal. This similarity does not, however, change the status of a person who is on a low-carb diet to a ketone diet.
- Carb Consumption: I will also emphatically state here that in both diets, there is a certainly a level of carb consumption. When people decide to engage in low carb diets or Ketogenic diet, they will still have to consume carbohydrate in one form or the other, and that is the similarity between the two diets.

- Protein and other Food Sources are consumed: In both diets, there is the intake of protein and other food sources. However, caution is recommended here when consuming protein because when it is high, it may hinder you from entering ketosis. We will discuss that more when we approach the short topic "How to Enter Ketosis Fast."

Starting the Ketogenic Diet Lifestyle

Starting Ketogenic lifestyle at the beginning of your diet requires you to know some important things. It is essential for you to understand that your fuel metabolism changes from carb to fat. Thus, as the river of carb dries up because you have cut it down from your food, your body makes an adjustment to burn an alternative fuel source which is fat, and it is broken down to ketones in the body. Your weight loss goal is achieved when you have fully entered into ketosis. In Ketosis, your body burns fat instead of conventional carb as a fuel source. But what does it take to make the change? Habit formations are one of your greatest aid. You need to develop a good habit that will help you stay in ketosis. While the cravings for carb might come down heavily upon you, you have to fight it off. A heavy loading of carb destroys your weight loss goal. Further down in this book, I will give you a Ketogenic kitchen list. It is good to have those food items in your pantry. Since the Ketogenic diet resolves around a full optimization of ketosis, I will give you some aid that will help you speed up your ketosis.

- Limit Carb Intake: One of the easiest and quickest ways to reach ketosis is by restricting carb intake per day to 20% of total calories. However, the higher you reduce the intake of carbs, the better. Some have lowered carb intake to 5% and got better results. To lower carbs, choose the fruits with low carb content and veggies with low carb content. Marinate them with healthy fats. Your blueberries or raspberries should be soaked in unsweetened coconut milk or heavy cream. And then your green veggies, broccoli, zucchini, and cauliflower should be covered with healthy olive oil or grass-fed butter.
- Incorporate Coconut Oil in Your Diet: Consuming coconut oil is one quick route to ketosis. Coconut Oil contains fats called medium-chain triglycerides (MCTs). The good thing about MCT is that unlike most fats, MCTs

are quickly absorbed and transported straight to the liver, where they are used quickly as converted energy or converted into ketones. Many are of the view that consuming coconut oil is one of the greatest ways to increase ketone levels in the lives of those afflicted with Alzheimer's disease and other nervous system diseases. Coconut oil has four basic types of MCTs. Fifty percent of the coconut oil is fat that is gotten from lauric acid. A higher percentage of lauric acid as suggested by many types of research produces a more sustainable level of ketosis. The reason for this is because it metabolizes slowly than other MCTs. In epileptic kids, MCTs have been used successfully to induce ketosis without limiting the number of carbs as it happens in a normal Ketogenic diet.

- Practice fasting: Intermittent fasting is a necessity if you want to speed up ketosis. Fasting is one of the fundamental weapons for getting into quick ketosis. Fasting can also be used to maintain ketosis since you are cutting down on calories and not eating protein or carbohydrate. Before you begin fasting, it is best to lower your carb for some few days before the fasting in order to avoid a hypoglycemic incident. It is easier to maintain ketosis if you are able to fast intermittently. As you undertake your fast, I recommend taking herbal teas and hydrating and taking organic coffee with MCT oil, or grass-fed butter or coconut oil. Ketone production is boosted by the small and medium chain fats, which goes a long way in stabilizing blood sugar more effectively than water fasting. Many people have reported excellent feelings while fasting.

- **Increase fat intake**: Eating plenty of healthy fat increases ketone levels and help you reach ketosis. A low carb keto diet not only reduces the level of carbs but very effective for weight loss, metabolic health and optimal exercise performance. When the Ketogenic diet is used for epilepsy treatment, it will be higher in fat percentage of about 85–90% of calories from fat. It is important to note that an increase in the consumption of fat does not necessarily mean a correspondent increase in ketone levels in the body system. Additionally, since the Ketogenic diet composes of a large percentage of fat, it is good when making the choice of fat to choose those that are high in quality. Such quality fat includes – coconut oil, lard, olive oil, avocado oil, butter, and tallow. Furthermore, high-fat foods that are very healthy yet low in carb content. However, for those whose main goal of engaging in the

Ketogenic diet is weight loss, you have to ensure that you are not consuming too many calories in total, as this may prevent your weight loss goals.

- **Obtain A ketone Meter:** The reason why you need a ketone meter to measure your ketosis is so that you know once you have entered ketosis the steps to take. It is important because there are many instruments out there. However, Ketone meters are the most effective and standard form of measuring your ketosis. However, it has one major problem. It is too expensive. A single ketone meter can cost up to $ 100, and the test per strip can be up to five bucks. The content of the meter includes a lancet pen, which is a device that jabs you in order to get blood. The meter beyond testing for ketones in your bloodstream, it also tests for glucose. The two most popular blood ketone meters on the market today – Precision Brand and

Nova Max. Both of them can be ordered from amzon.com. The problem with Nova Max as reported by many users is that it frequently gives you an error message and it does not give you any reading below 0.5 although their test strips are cheaper, precision strip gives you more accuracy with lesser error messages. Its drawback lies in the fact that it is much expensive per strips than Nova Max. One problem though it is that precision is not too effective on glucose measurement, but it measures ketones very effectively. However, if you want to decide which of the two products that you want to purchase, I will suggest that you read the reviews on amazon. This will help you make your mind up.

CHAPTER TWO

List of Persons Who can go on a Ketogenic Diet?

- Everybody can go on and lose weight rapidly. However, there are restrictions. The fundamental question is, can Ketogenic diet be undertaken by everybody? Are there people who are supposed to go on a Ketogenic diet or are there people who should not go on a Ketogenic diet? Let me try to make some list here.

- Pregnant and Breastfeeding Mom: A pregnant woman can go on a Ketogenic diet, but it must be carefully done with the guidance of a physician or dietitians. There is a risk for a pregnant woman. Serious weight loss at the time of pregnancy may affect the fetus or the baby because of the release of toxins. Weight loss during pregnancy and breastfeeding may have negative consequences for the baby or fetus as a result of the production of toxins by the fat cells. However, there is much research that encourages pregnant and breastfeeding moms to go on a Ketogenic diet.
- Type 1 Diabetes: In the case of type 1 diabetes, the body's defense system which can also be called the immune system assails a part of the body's pancreas. The reason why this happens is not known. The

body's immune system erroneously destroys the cells in the pancreas because it sees them as foreign. These cells which are destroyed by the immune system are known as islets, and they are the ones that are responsible for dictating the levels of glucose in the blood stream, and when they see that the level of glucose is high, they produce the amount of insulin required to bring blood sugar to normal levels. Without insulin, blood sugar can be really high, and a lot of devastating consequences can occur. I needed to explain this. Now, this is the catch when you are on a Ketogenic diet; there is a switch in the fuel source. Your body switches from burning carbs stored as glucose to fats. Since the intake of carb is limited, fat is used as a fuel source. Remember that at this stage your body is no longer taking in glucose. It will begin to break down the fat in the muscles and other parts of the body system. This happens when you are on a Ketogenic diet, and you have entered ketosis; what you use as energy is fat and it is the breakdown of this fat that results in the buildup of ketone bodies. Ketone bodies enter the blood stream, and a chemical imbalance occurs which is known as diabetic ketoacidosis. To engage in the Ketogenic diet without the direction of a physician is dangerous for Type 1 diabetes.

- Children: Kids can go on a Ketogenic Diet. Remember in the chronicle or history of Ketogenic diet we stated that one of the things that made it stage a good come back was when it was successfully administered on a kid to control his epilepsy in the 1990's.

- Elderly: Ketogenic diet is a diet that everyone can go on despite age categorization. It would, however, be advised that before the elderly decide to proceed on a Ketogenic diet, they consult their dietitians or physicians.

Benefits of Ketogenic Diet

We will discuss the benefits that can be obtained once you are on a Ketogenic diet. Once you are on a Ketogenic diet, these are the benefits that you will derive from being on a diet:

- **Epilepsy**: In the chronicles of Ketogenic diet, I have expounded with clarity how in the 1920s, the society heavily relied on a Ketogenic diet as a means of fighting epilepsy. Though drugs were to some extent effectively good, the diet was successfully dealing with epilepsy. It will be recalled that in 1994, the father of a kid who got tired of trying out conventional medicine because the seizure which his kid was having at that point defied any form of treatment. They had tried their hands on modern medicine, but failure hit them back at their faces. However, when they finally lay their hands on the Ketogenic diet, the kid was completely healed as long as he was on a diet. Beyond administering this diet on kids in those days, Ketogenic diet has successfully been tested on adults with amazing therapeutic results. Today, Ketogenic diet can handle epilepsy both in the young and adults.

- **Reversing Type 2 Diabetes**: This is one of the benefits of being on a Ketogenic diet. The many success stories of this diet which research has proven are that since the amount of carbohydrate that you take is lowered, then your blood sugar level is brought to the barest minimum. It is important to note that carb stimulates the body system to discharge the hormone called insulin. So when carb intake is lowered, the body does not release more insulin to control the blood sugar which will, in turn, increase the burning of fat that has been stored in the body. How then does this work in reversing Type 2 diabetes? The answer to the question is simple. The fundamental problem faced by people with diabetes is a high amount of blood sugar that comes primarily from carb intake. Once a person in on a Ketogenic diet, since he eats a fewer amount of carbs, the body can easily control the amount of blood sugar which has the capacity of reversing Type 2 diabetes.

- **Weight Loss**: What happens during ketosis? Your body switches from burning carbs as fuel into burning fat which results in tremendous weight loss. As you go deeper into the sea of ketosis, your body burns fat resulting in weight loss. Instead of other types of diets which many have been using for weight loss without success, with Ketogenic diet, you lose body fat and weight quickly.
- **Effective Mental Agility**: When ketosis mode is fully activated, there is a constant supply of ketones to the brain. Remember that when the body is not in ketosis mode and carb is steadily fed into the body system, the brain makes use of carb as a fuel source and many are of the opinion that mental activities and focus can be increased when more carbs are consumed. On the contrary, when you are fully in

ketosis, because your body makes a huge change in fuel consumption, meaning it burns more fat rather than the conventional carbs, fat in your body are broken down into ketone bodies. Other organs in the body can make use of fat. However, the brain makes use of ketones broken down from fat. During ketosis, there is usually increased the flow of ketone bodies to the brain giving it effective mental agility and focus.

- **Acne Reduction**: It is has been reported with huge success that many people who have acne problems when on low carb diet like the Ketogenic diet that acne is drastically reduced. When on a Ketogenic diet, the intake of carb is lowered. Where carbs are taken, the body needs to produce the hormone called insulin to reduce the amount of blood sugar in the blood stream. Acne is mostly caused and driven by insulin. It is the cornerstone of acne. Besides acting as the main agent that motivate skin cells to manufacture sebum (an oily secretion secreted by the sebaceous gland that lubricates the hair and skin that gives protection against bacteria) and keratin (a fibrous insoluble protein that is the main structural element in hair and nail), it heightens the secretion of many other hormones that causes acne. What does this all mean? When you are on a low carb diet like Ketogenic diet, the secretion of insulin to lower the amount of blood sugar in your blood stream is not necessarily needed since your body as a fat burning machine, does not need that. Insulin, being one of the fathers of acne, will be curtailed since you do not take many carbs that will summon its presence in your blood stream. When there is no sugar to reduce in the blood, I bet that insulin will continue sleeping.

- **Enhanced Stamina**: During the Ketogenic diet, your physical stamina and endurance will be enhanced since you will have access to storage of fat that your body has reserved. At a time of intense exercise, your stored carbs will melt away like the dissolving ice beaten by summer light within a couple of hours. On the other hand, your fat storage can last longer than your carbs. When you are carb adapted, your fat stores are easily depleted during a short time of intense exercise and to refill; you must keep eating. However, when you are on a Ketogenic diet, most of the fuel that is available is fat with long lasting effects than your regular carb stores. The body and your brain are energized by your fat stores making you last longer in exercise and have a lot of stamina than someone who is relying on carbs for his stamina and endurance.

- **Enhanced Performance**: Since your body is experiencing a shift from what it is used to, it is possible that at the formative stage of the Ketogenic diet, you might experience some form of reduced performance. But will this remain for a long time? Certainly no. The benefits of going Ketogenic are more long term than short term. Today, there are many athletes that are going Ketogenic and have seen very effective and great performances especially in long distance running. As I have explained earlier, your fat stores last longer than your carb stores. Since fat stores last longer, an athlete can perform for a prolonged period without refueling with external energy.

- **Decreased Aging**: With Ketogenic diet, your body can maintain a very nice look. When you have entered ketosis, ketone bones are produced. These bodies may decrease the aging process by blocking a group of enzymes known as Histone Deacetylases. The enzymes function to keep a couple of genes known as Forkhead box O3 and Metallothionein 2A turned off. These genes can empower other cells to resist oxidative stress. The good thing is that the ketone bodies produce when a full fledge ketosis has been entered can block Forkhead box O3 allowing the genes to be reactivated which prevents oxidative stress because it is this oxidative stress that indirectly causes aging. Besides, the Ketogenic diet reduces blood sugar levels. It is important to know that when sugar levels are reduced, glycation and the production of enhanced glycation by-product materials made from high blood sugar heightens tissue damage, diabetes, and aging. Finally, Ketogenic diet is a catalyst that reduces triglycerides which are known for causing a lot of terminal diseases.

- **Alzheimer disease**: This is a mental disorder that causes dementia because of the progressive degradation of the brain. One of the features of this disease is a decreasing ability of the brain to metabolize glucose. Whenever the brain is unable to metabolize glucose, it can have a lot of impact on the brain. However, with ketone bodies when a person is fully into ketosis, the supply of ketones to the brain when on a Ketogenic diet reduces the brain over dependence on glucose.

How to Measure Ketosis

- **Urine Test**: This is one way to measure your ketones for the purpose of ascertaining whether you are in ketosis. Using urine strips, you can easily and simply determine your ketosis without much cost. Testing your urine will readily reveal to you if you have gone over the rooftop by eating higher than recommended carbs. Once you dip the stick into your urine, it will turn purple indicating the presence of ketones in your body. A good result for the presence of ketones is dark purple color. When no precise color is shown, it means that you might not have entered ketosis yet.
- **Obtain a ketone Meter**: Ketone meters are the most effective and standard form of measuring your ketosis. However, it has one major problem. It is too

expensive. A single ketone meter can cost up to $ 100, and the test per strip can be up to five bucks. The content of the meter includes a lancet pen, which is a device that jabs you in order to get blood. The meter beyond testing for ketones in your bloodstream, it also tests for glucose. The two most popular blood ketone meters on the market today – Precision Brand and Nova Max. Both of them can be ordered from amzon.com. The problem with Nova Max as reported by many users is that it frequently gives you an error message and it does not give you any reading below 0.5 although their test strips are cheaper, Precision Brand strip gives you more accuracy with lesser error messages. Its drawback lies in the fact that it is expensive per strips than Nova Max. One problem though it is that precision is not too effective on glucose measurement, but it measures ketones very effectively. However, if you want to decide which of the two products that you want to purchase, I will suggest that you read the reviews on amazon. This will help you make your mind up.

- **Ketone Breath Analysers**: Measuring your breath through the breath ketone analyzers is a good way of knowing whether you have fully entered into ketosis. They are very expensive, and they can be ordered from Amazon. However, they are less expensive than the blood ketone meters. They come in two forms – disposable and reusable. The results of these tests come in different form. They will not give you an accurate result of what the level of your blood ketones is but rather display for you an array of colors. It is not a form of yes or no. It will either give this color for positive that you are in ketosis or that color for negative that you are not in ketosis. All the same, when you measure your blood ketones with ketone breath analyzers, the yellow and tan are indicators that the result is negative that you have not yet entered ketosis. When the result shows you pink or purple, it means that you are fully into ketosis. One major problem as complained by users of these breath analyzers is their inaccuracy. Sometimes, the results obtained are not true. Besides that, I will not encourage anyone who is just starting a Ketogenic diet to use the breath analyzers. Blood ketone meters are by far the best since they give you a much accurate result. If you are a seasoned dieter on Ketone, you can try this breath analyzer since the chances are that you are following your diet right. You know what you want. However, for beginners, it is good to use the blood ketone meters. Besides, the instructions for usage on the disposable has been reported to be complex, and unless carefully used, mistakes abound.

How to Know When You Have Entered Ketosis

The fundamental goal of being on a Ketogenic diet is to enter ketosis in which case your body makes a huge switch from a carb burning machine into a fat burning machine, and that is actually where the weight loss begins. How do you know that you have entered ketosis for your Ketogenic diet to be effective? How do you know that you are fully into ketosis for an optimum weight loss which is the basis for being on a diet? There are many of those signs, and I will explain them here.

Excessive thirst and sometimes feeling dry in the mouth. When you feel thirst and excessive dryness in the mouth, you might have entered ketosis. It is important for you to take a lot of liquids such as water and salt so that you can obtain a lot of electrolytes to resolve this.

Frequent urination. Ketone bodies are produced when you are fully into ketosis. One of the ketones that are produced is called acetoacetate, whose end is in your urine. For most beginners on the Ketogenic diet, it is possible to experience frequent visits to the bathroom. Do not be alarmed; it could be that you have entered ketosis.

The low rate of hunger. This is the evidence of many people who are on a Ketogenic diet. The reason for this is diverse. When you are in ketosis, your body uses its fat stores for fuel. Again, due to a high fraction of protein and vegetable intake and the changes experienced by your hunger hormones could cause that. Additionally, when the urge for eating does not come more frequently, the possibility is that you are in ketosis.

Your breath is another fundamental index for dictating that you are in ketosis. As you entered ketosis, it is possible that your breath takes on a fruity texture. The reason for this is because of ketone bodies being passed through your breath. The particular ketone that is responsible for that is called acetone. Brush your teeth as many times a day that you can afford to do to avoid fruity breath. If that is what you are currently experiencing, then I congratulate you because it is possible that you have entered ketosis. However, this bad breath is transient and not permanent. As your time in the diet enlarges, the fruity breath goes away on its own.

Rapid weight loss. To lose weight rapidly, then Ketogenic diet is your solution. And that is one of the things you will experience once you have entered ketosis. Most people undergo rapid weight loss in their first week of dieting this is because a lot of your fat stores are being used plus carbs and water in your body system are being utilized by your body system.

Energetic strength. The level of energy you feel in your body will increase. Your fat stores are being used up during this process and fat in your body is readily broken down. Before this stage is attained, at the early stages of dieting, it is possible to have a Keto flu. This is because your body at that period is working very hard to adjust to the new fuel source. Some people feel tiredness, feeling sick and other types of feelings. As you age in the diet, all of these feelings will disappear. You will begin to feel strengthened and energetic.

The increased presence of ketones in the blood. As your blood sugar levels reduce, something else fills your blood stream – ketones. When you gather more distance in the diet, you will be burning mainly fat and ketones as your fuel source.

Improved mental focus. At the start of the Ketogenic diet, your body makes an adaptation from burning carbs to burning fat. When you entered into ketosis, your brain begins to burn ketones instead of glucose gotten from carbs. So when you begin to experience improved mental focus, it is one of the indexes of ketosis.

Tiredness and exhaustion. When making a switch from carbs to Ketogenic diet, many dieters face a lot of issues. At the early phase of dieting, many feel tired and exhausted. This is because of the initial change in the fuel source. However, if endured, the long-term benefits of Ketogenic are more than the reactions that your body feels. Feelings of tiredness and exhaustion are symptoms of ketosis.

Digestion during the beginning period of the dieting on a Ketogenic diet may be a problem. Depending on your body system, this is not common to everyone. Some experience constipation. This is however limited to the transitional phase of the diet. The moment you are fully transitioned, this will stop. This may also be an indication of ketosis. As I said, people's experience on the Ketogenic diet varies. Yours might not be the same with that of another.

Sleeplessness is another index that ketosis has been entered. This experience is usually for those who first start out on a diet. A change of diet for some has been associated with insomnia. Nevertheless, this does not last for long as it soon disappears within a short time.

Part 2

CHAPTER THREE

The Keto Lifestyle

Ketogenic or Keto lifestyle is a dieting lifestyle of curtailing the intake of high carbohydrate based food. Keto dieting encourages consumption of high fat food and low protein base food. Ketogenic dieting aims at putting the body into the state of *"Ketosis."* In Ketosis, excess fat is converted into *"Ketones"* in the liver which is used as the source of energy for the body in place of carbohydrate. Keto dieting program aims at transforming the body into a fat burning machine.

What to Eat During Ketogenic Diet

Planning is very important for every Ketogenic diet that you decide to go on because the diet works on recognized principles without the observance of which, quick weight loss might not be attained. The amount of food you eat, the type of food you eat will either delay your ketosis or hinder it completely. The less quantity of carbs you eat, let us say 18 to 20 grams daily, the better your chances of getting into ketosis and if you decided to narrow it down to 15 grams, the better your chances of entering into the state of ketosis within a short time. The recommended intake of carbs in a proper Ketogenic diet is within the range of 20 percent to 30 percent. However, to get better results, it is good if you can lower your carb intake. For your nutrients, it is recommended that it should be 70 percent, fats should be 25 percent, and your carbs should be 5 percent. Your nutrient intake can also be structured in this form, 70% fats, 25% protein, and 5% carbohydrate. The source of your carbs should be mostly obtained from veggies, dairy products, and nuts. I have listed some nutritious food that you can eat.

- Meat: Here you can eat lamb, beef, pork, etc.
- Eggs: They are very rich in fat content.
- Cheese: Make sure that they do not contain carbs

- Veggies: They contain some amount of carbs but make sure that what you eat is not too rich in carbs, vegetables like cabbage and lettuce are okay.
- Nuts: They are a good source of low carbs especially walnut and almonds.

However, always eat your nut with a sense of moderation not to blow your carb intake over the top.

What Not to Eat

There are certain food products which you must avoid if you want to have a good result from your Ketogenic diet. The majority of your meal should be protein and vegetables. Never eat starchy carbs like bread, pasta, cereals, potatoes, beans, legumes or some fruits. They will hinder the whole process of your Ketogenic diet and can stop you from getting into ketosis.

Why You Need A Diet Plan?

The Ketogenic diet is built on a strong foundation of healthy foods that help achieve weight loss effortlessly. If you carefully prepare a meal plan, it will prevent you from ordering takeout. This diet will then culture you into a habit that will eliminate completely the desire for processed foods which will, in turn, help you to lead the healthy life and attain weight loss without a struggle.

Knowledge is information and others called it power. And that is true. If you look at some of the shopping list mentioned in this book, you will notice that it will help you to become an informed shopper who knows the healthy foods to buy that will give him the best result in eating foods which will help your Ketogenic diet. When you shop by yourself, the shopping educates you in buying food items that are necessary for your ketone diet which will, in the end, give you healthy appearance and make your weight loss aim a reality.

He who fails to plan they say plans to fail. Having a meal plan will save you a lot of money. In this book, we have covered the low dollar Ketogenic diet and how it will help you to cut down on the cost of your Ketogenic diet. If you plan well, the meal plan will let you know what you need to purchase which will, in the long run, reduce cost.

If you want to lead the Ketogenic diet life, then know that it is time-consuming. You will have to spend time cooking, and this is where it can get boring at times. Sometimes, thinking of cooking alone can be a challenging mountain to climb. This is where having a meal plan helps a lot. Once your meal is planned out, you will just go straight ahead to cook your food and save yourself the time you waste on thinking what am I to cook.

The good thing about the Ketogenic diet is that you do not need to count the calories that you take per meal. However, for those who still want to know the exact amount of nutrient that they are consuming, a prepared meal plan is just the right thing you need.

With your meal plan, you are able to know what exactly to eat and the amount of calorie content in each diet.

How to Enter Ketosis Fast

There are practical ways to ensure that you enter into ketosis within a short time. It is when you do this that you will enter into ketosis within a short time. It all depends on how fast you want to get into ketosis. Below are some of the things that you can do in order to ensure that ketosis mode is activated.

Reduce Carb Intake: to achieve ketosis; you need to restrict the amount of carbohydrate that you consume to 20 grams per day. The intake of 20 grams per day is the recommended amount of carbs that you need for fully optimized ketosis and effective Ketogenic diet.

However, you need to understand that the lesser carb you absorb into your system, the quicker your ketosis. It is important for you to understand that your ketosis activation is strictly in your hands. Always remember that the lesser the amount of carbs that you intake, the faster you get into ketosis.

Reduce Protein Intake: Before you enter into Ketosis, one thing you need to know is that you will have to keep an eye on your protein intake. It should never be above 50 grams to 100 grams for ladies and for men, it should be about 70 grams of protein daily. If you ingest that amount of protein and found out that after some days, you have not still entered into ketosis, then you will have to cut it further down. Why do you need to keep an eye on your protein intake? Now, if you consume excess protein than what your body requires, the body converts this protein into glucose. This will hinder you from getting into ketosis because you have glucose in your body and the organs will rather make use of it than embark on using fat as a fuel source. It is only when glucose intake is restricted whether through protein converted to glucose or through carbs that you will enter ketosis fully. The ball is in your hands, and you can kick it however you desire.

Increase Fat Intake: to have an effective ketosis within the shortest possible time; fat must constitute at least above 70 percent of your calories. Eat more of Hollandaise, Avocado, egg yolk, olives, meat, pork, etc. You can also get fat from this variety of products:

1. Chicken fat

2. Coconut oil

3. Grass-fed butter

4. Peanut oil

5. Grass fed beef tallow

6. Lard gotten from pigs

7. Organic and pastured chicken Eggs

8. Palm oil

Watch your Snack Intake: Too much of snack can hinder you from entering into full ketosis within the shortest time.

Irregular Fasting: The attainment of ketosis is something you must learn to build up with time. In some other situations, fasting will help you to enter into ketosis faster. This is something you must do by yourself. When you have achieved full ketosis status, then this becomes the natural thing that will be happening to you. This is because as you get into full ketosis, you will experience a steady washing away of your desire to eat. What do I mean? It means that when you have entered into ketosis on a Ketogenic diet, you will notice a reduction of your appetite. The occurrence of this may take time, but it will surely happen. Skipping breakfast or dinner will be of immense help as it will hasten your entrance into the door of ketosis.

Forming Good Habit: Achieving ketosis within the shortest time is easy but impossible without the development of good habit pattern. Without discipline, it is impossible to achieve full blown ketosis status. Sometimes, you will be magnetized by your regular carb diet. They may sometimes be too tempting to resist, and it will want to oppose Ketogenic diet and close the gate of ketosis from opening to you. You know the rules, eat your daily 20 grams of carb per day and your high fat of 70 to 80 percent. Your protein intake should be about 70 grams or lesser not more than that. It is a discipline which you have to learn. When the desire for high carb diet is burning intensely in you, the first thing to do is to ensure that you eat some nuts especially those that are very low in carbs like walnut. It is this habit that if well-formed will help you in entering ketosis in time and maintain that state.

Beyond doubt, the reservoir of knowledge that you have has been increased as it regards Ketogenic diet. If we stop at this point, it will be a dwarf understanding of Ketogenic diet. We have made huge progress so far since beginning this book, and it seems that one important thing has not been discussed yet. It is therefore highly imperative that we further this knowledge. We will be discussing something that is fundamental. Before you enter into a full ketosis mode, your body like a computer is initializing. It is taking some important steps towards entering into ketosis. Please permit my use of language in making reference to a computer. However, when full ketosis mode is activated, what are the reactions that you will experience within your body. It is this body reaction to a Ketogenic diet that many categorize as the disadvantages of Ketogenic diet. How do you also measure ketosis? We will be paying attention to some of these reactions and measurement of ketosis.

For the purposes of emphasis, the Ketogenic diet plan is more effective when your body gets into ketosis where your body switches from a carb burning machine to a fat burning machine. As this happens, the end products that are generated are called ketones. These ketones come out through the breath when it takes on a fruity dimension, urine, and even sweat. In effect, by testing your urine, it is possible to know whether you are in ketosis. The question is how do I measure my ketones level? I will say here that if you desire to measure it, it is a matter of set goals. You should not allow measuring ketones to become your primary consuming passion. You will get into ketosis, and you will lose weight, but do not pay too much attention to it so that you will begin to worry much.

Common Challenges of Ketogenic dieters

The Ketogenic diet has come under severe attack in the recent years with many saying that there is no scientific basis for the diet. Nevertheless, I have given you the scientific proof of the diet in this book. Beyond that, many people have had success stories from this diet from weight loss to a healthy life. The diet has its own challenges. There are difficulties and challenges that you will experience. It may be different, but they are challenges that you can triumph.

Products Labels

Although I have suggested buying all of your products directly from the farmers market near you for effective Ketogenic diet, there are certain circumstances that will require you buying from the store. This is to ensure that what you are buying is organic. If you have to buy anything that is organic from the store, then make sure that you read every label carefully. I suggest making a thorough check of your item to find the best Ketogenic diet product. Buying your veggies and other stuff from the farmers market near you is the best thing that can happen to you. However, where you cannot buy directly from the farmers market near your area, make sure that you check the product's label very carefully. If you do not do this, it is possible to buy foods that are high in carb content.

Indecision

Sometimes your body might want to tempt you into the state of unpreparedness. It may want to keep you in a permanent cycle of indecision, "I will soon begin my diet." The word soon keeps happening to you until it gets to a point when you will lose complete and total interest in the diet. Never wait for the perfect time for you to start your Ketogenic diet. It is possible to feel completely unprepared for the necessary change. Some people are stuck in an everlasting chain of research. "I need to know this before I begin my diet." Don't get stuck in that. Change is something that is not comfortable to make, and if you keep searching for excuses, then it is possible not to begin the diet at all.

Diet Apathy

The Ketogenic diet is indeed a fun-filled from the beginning to the end. Will this remain so until the end? If you log onto any of the social media, be it Instagram, Twitter, or even Facebook, you will be over flooded with people's good days that gives you a perfect interest about the diet. Nevertheless, the bad days are coming, and when they come, you have to learn to make it exciting. The veterans in the diet have their bad days when Ketogenic diet food becomes boring. During that time, the temptation to return to the old fashion of eating is usually strong. Do not let these feelings take control of you. Rather, you should control them. Sometimes the feelings of resentment, frustration, tiredness, with cooking becoming a chore. When you experience these times, know that it is normal. It happens. Acknowledge this and give yourself space to feel it, and try to get over it. I recommend strongly having a meal plan so that you can have different things to eat on different days. It adds interest and kills apathy. At such times, you can also seek the advice of other dieters on how they overcame their bad days. Belong to a forum and join a community of Ketogenic dieters. It will help you in the days of diet struggles.

Strange Reactions

The moment you change your normal diet to a Ketogenic diet, some persons in your life will begin to express their own insecurities and fears. You will notice this through their comments. They will not stop there, and they will make additional comments if you lose more weight. Many will tell you how they can never give up their carb foods. Should that border you? No. You have chosen the path of healthy eating, be proud to walk through it. The opinion of people and what they think should not hinder you. Just know that not everybody will be comfortable with the way that you eat. That is the reason why you should be meticulous with people who are your friends. Many of them might discourage you. People who will understand and reason with you can be a great source of encouragement to you.

Part 3

CHAPTER FOUR

Shopping Tips for Ketogenic Diet

You have read how to do a low dollar Ketogenic diet, but unless you know some shopping tips, it is possible to spend more on your diet making it uncomfortable for you to continue dieting. Shopping! With its many beautiful and eye, magnetizing shelves that are loaded with goods can become the place where you spend a lot of money. For Ketogenic dietary purposes, always buy food items from the farmers market near you.

Shop for Mostly Organic Foods

Foods in their natural state are the best for Ketogenic diet. Many of the foods that have been refined have had their nutrients washed away through the process of refinement. They mostly lack the essential nutrients that you need. Shop wisely.

Follow the Principles of Time

The best time to shop as I have recommended in the low dollar Ketogenic diet is to do it after evening meals. However, you have to strike a balance between evening meals and rush hour. This is because rushing up to purchase things could make you miss the important details on labels of food products. If you rush, the chances are that you may not read products label well.

It may read "zero carbs" or "carb free" but it contains carb. Besides, if it is rush hour shopping, the queues are normally longer. Frustration can build. Grocery shopping is an important thing that you need some level of focus to do effectively. This is because what you are buying can affect your health and the health of your family too. If it can affect them, then it is something you should not rush.

Carefully Study Your Shopping Aisle

Some of the aisles where you see cheap products might have some of the healthiest foods. So do not ignore them. Arm yourself with a shopping list and thoroughly search them. Do not overlook them because they can give you some healthy foods that you need.

Study Carefully the Ingredients Details

It is fundamental for effective shopping to read the ingredients that are contained in a product that you want to buy. If the ingredient contains what will hinder your Ketogenic diet, then put it down. If you buy ingredients that are high in carb, then you are likely not to lose weight rapidly.

Small Cart for Cutting Expenses

Except if you are going for a bulk purchase or you are using a coupon, it is wise to pick a small cart or basket that is available to you. Why do you need to do that? This will help you make wise purchases. The smaller the cart, the fewer items that you are likely to purchase. However, if you decide to pick up a trolley and glide it across different aisles, I can assure you that you are likely to purchase products for your Ketogenic diet, which you have at home.

Refrigerated Products

Some of the veggies that you will purchase may be frozen. Does that mean that they are bad? No. These veggies are still as nutritious as the fresh ones. The Jerusalem artichokes, carrots and brussels sprouts are still fresh and important even though they may look frozen.

Pay Cash

You may be thinking that buying your products on credits is more efficient for your shopping. Many people who go to the grocery store to buy food products purchase more junk and processed foods. So unless you are short of cash, buy the product and pay in cash. In addition, if you want to buy on credit, then do not buy junk food. If you buy junk and processed foods; your rapid weight loss will not be achieved

Change Your Shopping Time

This is sound wisdom. Many Americans prefer shopping on Saturdays and Sundays. During those weekends, where most people are not busy, the grocery store is filled with people. Avoid that. This is the attitude of most Americans. You can change your shopping time to Tuesday if you are free or Fridays. Depending on how relaxed your schedules are. Then your Saturdays will be for cooking your diet meals. I have said it that if you want to cut down the cost of your Ketogenic diet, then you must learn to prepare everything by yourself. Beyond that, for people with children who are employed, you can use your weekend to prepare your meals and refrigerate them. Then from Monday to Fridays, you put your foods in a bag and head to your job. Just make sure that you cook different foods during the weekend so that you do not get bored with eating the same meal.

Watch Out For Fancy Labels

Have you realized that products that are more expensive come in fancy packages? A study has found that food suppliers employ the use of fancy fonts and labels as an excuse for their high price. The research had further stated that people tend to think that they will get more value for their money from fancy and attractive product labels.

Avoid Prepared Food Sections

Have you seen the prepared food sections of many grocery stores in the country? It has experienced tremendous growth in recent years because many in America are looking for alternatives to expensive restaurants. In 2011, the supermarket restaurants in the USA grew to 14 billion dollars. Why? The reason for this is clear. Many Americans are looking for alternatives to lower cost of food. However, you need to understand that if you want to lower the cost of your Ketogenic diet, you must make a conscious effort to go for your shopping alone and avoid eating in the supermarket restaurants. Now combine this tip with low dollar Ketogenic diet, and you will cut the cost of dieting to the lowest form.

Buy Un-Popular Brand

Stay on the shelf or die! Many big manufacturers in America are using all forms of malpractices to keep small manufacturers out of the shelf. Independent Marketers in California sued Sara Lee for paying supermarkets so that their products are at the bottom of the shelf. However, some of this unknown brand have the healthiest foods than the famous brands.

Low Dollar Ketogenic diet

Many people starting out the Ketogenic diet are not aware of how expensive it is. They will not understand this until their bills increased ten times over. That is when they will begin to complain that the diet is too expensive and they cannot continue with it. For best Ketogenic diet, most of your foods will be organic. In the grocery store, some of the most expensive food products in the store are organic foods. This, therefore, means that anyone who wants to do the Ketogenic diet must be ready to spend money on his diet. However, I will tell you how you can be on a diet and still spend a little amount of money.

Prioritization

This is the first place to begin your Ketogenic diet. You have to make a decision on what is more important. The Ketogenic diet lifestyle requires this decision. There are certain things that are not important that steadily drain down dollars from your wallet. I will leave that decision to you. Nevertheless, what if the money spent on some of the pleasurable things in your life can be given up and devoted to your diet? Setting your priorities right is important. Spend money on things that are important to you. Your pleasurable sports can be limited to feed your Ketogenic diet bill. If the things that are in your life right now are things of necessity, then that is good and excellent. Many people are murmuring about the expensiveness of the Ketogenic diet. However, they have many fancy things that pile up bills. A life lived in health when the money is spent on this diet by far outweighs being an ever present guest in a hospital or even buying expensive health care insurance. The food you eat has a direct link to your health.

Avoid Waste

Let nothing be wasted! It will help you to cut down cost. This is the most efficient way to manage resources. For instance, the bones you have used are not to be discarded; you can reuse them for making another set of broth. The pan drippings you have used can be reserved for future usage. For your fresh produce, employ wisdom. Do not waste it. Cut just about what you need. Throw nothing away.

This is the biggest problem of dieters – whether they are veteran dieters or beginners. Food wastage will draw many holes in your wallet and finances. Your leftovers should not be a bosom friend of the dustbin. It should be frozen in the refrigerator to be used again. A food saver will help you to save money. Your vegetables may not look freshly appetizing from 3 days ago, but they are still delicious with nutritional value. So don't waste any of your food. It will make your low dollar Ketogenic diet a reality.

Direct Farmers Purchase

The farmers market that is near you is a great source of fresh and inexpensive food. Once you identify yourself with the local farmers around you, it will amaze you the amount of money that you will save when you have a personal relationship with the local farmers, and you begin to buy fresh produce directly from them. As you devote your loyalty to them by making regular purchases, they will give you items like bones and organs at a discount. Besides that, after a hot farming day, many farmers are constrained by situations to sell their farm produce so that it does not waste. The farmers may be willing to sell their produce at a cheaper rate.

Buy Food Items Nearing Expiring Date

The best time to go for grocery shopping is just before your evening meal. Meats and items that are nearing their expiry date are heavily discounted. Do not be alarmed; they are good for consumption.

Buy in Bulk

One of the easiest ways to save money is to purchase your food items in bulk. For instance, a bag of chicken in a nearby store around you can be $ 10 and can last you almost a week. For those who want to shop online, check for Grassland Beef that can be shipped to your house in a frozen box. The great thing about bulk buying is that it gives a discount that you will not be able to get if you buy your items one after the other. If the goods that you want to purchase are seasonal goods, then during the season make your purchases in large quantity. If you buy in bulk, you can preserve the freshness of your product by either freezing, fermenting or other methods of preservation that is best suited to you.

Personally, make your stuff

If you buy everything you need for your Ketogenic diet, it will increase your expenses. However, if make your own flavor, your spending on a diet will be little. Prepare your homemade stock and other condiments that you make by yourself. This will reduce expenses.

Let this be a discipline that you will learn every time by making your own stuff from scratch. What you need if you want to make everything yourself are the basic ingredients.

Effective Budget Planning

When you plan a budget, it will help you to keep an eye on what, where and which things are needed to be purchased. It will empower you to keep away from ostentatious purchases that pile up the mountains and the hills of bills. Expensive snacks and desserts that increase your spending should be avoided through effective budget planning.

Adopt Simple Meal Plans

Keep everything simple. Prepare most of your meals using cheap items for your diet. The simpler, the better as this will cut down your spending a lot.

Cultivate a Garden

For those who love gardening, you have an added advantage towards lowering the cost of your Ketogenic diet meals. With a tiny amount of $2 invested in each plant, it will surprise you at a number of plants that you will produce from your homemade garden. Thinking of how to begin, all you need is a windowsill for your herb garden which will give you fresh herbs from your home directly.

Plan Ahead

To be successful in your Ketogenic diet by lowering cost, then planning is your number one key. If you plan your meals ahead of time, you will reduce cost. It all depends on your personal preference and style. While others can cook food from available ingredients, yet for some, they need planning in order to be effective. So style your cooking according to what you know that you can do. Planning for some people is an indispensable tool while others need not make a plan to avoid wastage. It is possible that your plan may change from one day to another. If you want to preserve your own food, it is highly important that the leftovers food that has a short lifespan such as berries and vegetables are eaten within few days after consumption.

Costco Membership

Aimed at cutting down the cost of your Ketogenic diet, then you may consider Costco membership or any membership at your local food store or market. Although I will always suggest buying all your Ketogenic diet recipes directly from the farmers market available near you, it does not that mean that those who are not able to buy directly from the farmers market cannot do the Ketogenic diet. The answer is no. If you can't buy directly from the market, then I will suggest getting a Costco membership card. The membership card for gold card owners will cost you an amazing $ 55 per year. There is another membership card that cost $ 110 per year. Depending on your financial weight, you can get a membership card and enjoy a lot of discounts. A complete rotisserie chicken will cost you $ 5, and they are very big, and two dozen of eggs cost just $ 3. There are other inexpensive items when purchased in bulk such as oils, nuts, avocado, meat, and cheese. You can also buy your items at Costco in bulk. This will help you to save a lot of money and cut down the cost of your Ketogenic diet. If you live in the UK, Costco in London is three – Chingford, Thurrock, and Wardford. If you live in Germany, you can find Costco in Berlin, Frankfurt, and Hussen. In Australia, you can find Costco in Docklands, Canberra, Auburn, and Adelaide. Besides that, you can do a simple Google search of Costco near you.

Coupons, Gifts, and Discounts

There are many coupons for your Ketogenic diet food items in many grocery stores around you. If you decide to use them, you will reduce the cost of your diet. With the abundance of android apps, many of them can give you coupons that you can use for purchasing keto food items. Many stores are willing to offer you a reward for your loyalty with a coupon or a membership card. With your membership card, you can get special offers for food items and in some cases home delivery services. Even online stores offer coupons. You can use them to make your purchases and get discounts.

Use a Dehydrator

The use of a refrigerator is a great idea for the preservation of food items. However, beyond the use of a refrigerator, a dehydrator can be used to preserve your food items. Sometimes, the store offers more for sale than the space in your refrigerator. You may want to use the opportunity to buy more meat since they are sold at a discount price. Dehydrate the meat and store it for future use. If you have a garden and your garden produces a lot of foods than you need, your refrigerator being full, your dehydrator can be used to preserve the foods that can be used in the future.

Purchase during Seasonal Availability

Veggies from the farmers market are seasonal. This means that there are times when they will be cheaper because it is their seasons. Although this will never be the case for you if you make your purchases from the stores, you will only notice it when it is not the season in their prices. It will be slightly more expensive when it is the beginning of their seasons since it is not available in large quantity. Due to increased growth of technology and the prevalence of preservation machinery, stores around the world can offer food items at any time of the year. It is not uncommon to see fresh strawberries in the month of February or even pumpkin during the month of June on the shelves of many grocery stores, but because it is the store and you make these purchases at your convenience, it will cost you more.

Search for Cheaper Suppliers near You

You may want to make a list of suppliers whose products and services are cheaper in your location. This will help you to cut down the cost of your Ketogenic diet. Categorize your suppliers. Know those whose meat and animal products are cheaper, your baking essentials, veggies and fruits, sweeteners, nuts and seeds, berries and spices. Find out those who offer the cheaper sale of eggs, fruits, and chicken. If you are in Canada or UK or Germany or Australia, you can take your search to the internet and look for the available store that sells cheap stuff. It will help you to cut down the cost of your Ketogenic diet.

Prepare a Shopping List

Thinking of hitting the road to the store for shopping, always prepare a shopping list. Have a piece of paper or an iPad or android apps for your shopping list preparation. The advantage of this is to ensure that you know the product that you want to purchase so that you do not go and buy things you might not need.

Buy Inexpensive Ketogenic Diet Recipes

Have you seen the price of organic recipes in the store? Expensive huh? Yes, they are and to lower the cost of your Ketogenic diet, buy inexpensive recipes. Buy simple recipes like meat, seasonal veggies, nuts, and cheese.

Purchase Cheaper Meat Cut

There are many cheaper types of meat cut out there. For effective cooking of meat cuts, make use of a pressure cooker or slow cooker. It will cook the meat for you so that it can fall apart. Marrow bones and offal with their high nutrient contents are usually cheaper than other cuts.

Know What Beef to Buy

Grass-fed or pastured or grain-fed beef? Which of these will cut down the cost of your Ketogenic diet? Grass fed animals are those animals that have been feeding on grass for their whole life. Can animals that fed grass and during winter silage be called grass fed? No. They are not. They are rather pastured-fed animals. Grain fed meat from animals that have been in confinement should be avoided. However, buy the one that you can afford to purchase employing all the methods discussed above for lowering the cost of your purchases.

Eat Dessert Occasionally

Ketogenic diet desserts are many. The Desserts may look so wonderful, but it may add to the expenses of your diet. It is sound wisdom to eat dessert occasionally in order to cut down the cost of your diet. Though delicious, the more treats you eat, the more expensive your diet will be. If you want to cut costs, these desserts should infrequently be eaten and should not be daily affairs except you do not want to live the low the dollar Ketogenic diet lifestyle.

Part 4

CHAPTER FIVE

Introduction

One of the reasons why the Ketogenic diet has gained a lot of acceptance today is because of its ability to help many dieters achieve quick and a rapid weight loss. Where other forms of diet have failed, the Ketogenic diet has triumphed. That is why it has achieved many laurels of successes as seen in the acceptance that it has obtained so far even among dietitians, physicians, and dieters. By restricting the intake of carbs which end product is glucose, you set yourself on a course of having your body change from burning glucose for energy to burning fat. This change in body usage of fuel comes when the dieter enters into ketosis. It is during ketosis that ketone bodies are produced due to the consistent body breakdown of stored fat. Having stated that, does Ketogenic diet has any therapeutic benefit? Many researchers in recent years have surfaced showing that Ketogenic diet can be used to cure multiple diseases. If you recall, one of the main reasons why this diet gathered a lot of acceptance in the society today is its cure or regulation of epilepsy. But today, it has extended its frontiers from epilepsy to many other therapeutic remedies. Beyond this, it is important to highlight some of the withdrawal symptoms likely to be encountered when a dieter decides to stop the

Ketogenic diet. Why am I doing that? I do not want you to begin to worry thinking that something has happened to your health. Let us now look at some of the medical benefits of Ketogenic diet which dieters are more likely to benefit from.

Medical Effects of Ketogenic Diet

A lot of scientific research has been conducted that have discovered a lot of elements in Ketogenic diets with varied therapeutic benefits. I will make a list of them for you. Here they are:

- Epilepsy
- Alzheimer Disease
- Parkinson Disease
- Cancer

- Diabetes
- Autism
- Migraine
- Acne
- Reduction of blood sugar and insulin
- Reduce blood pressure
- Cure for many brain disorders
- Anti-aging
- Amyotrophic Lateral Sclerosis
- Stroke
- Cure for Mitochondrial Disorder
- Cure for Brain Trauma

From the above list, it can be seen that the health benefits of Ketogenic diet are numerous. Do you know anyone or family members suffering from the above-listed diseases, then your solution lies in this diet. Put them on it and see a remarkable improvement in their health status.

Withdrawal Symptoms of Ketogenic Diet

- Many Ketogenic diet books will never tell you this because they are trying to sell their books to you and make sure that you buy it. But I have decided that beyond selling this book to you, I am giving you a much vital information that will help you anytime you decided to put a pause on the Ketogenic diet for a while. The burning question is, what will happen when you eventually stop the Ketogenic diet and returned back to your normal diet or change to other forms of low carb diets?

- We will consider some of these factors, and I will tell you what you can do in order to maintain your weight after stopping the Ketogenic diet.
- Weight Gain: We have stated somewhere in this book that Ketogenic diet is a fast weight loss diet that enables dieters to lose weight with unimaginable speed. While this is true and an established fact, there are many things that will happen to you once you want to withdraw from the Ketogenic diet. One of it is weight gain. You were on a low-carb diet that helped you burnt down fat. However, when you stop the Ketogenic diet, it is possible to gain back all the weight that you have lost. When you stop Keto, and you go back to your old eating habit, you will gain back all the weight that you have lost. If you continue eating just the way that you desire, it is possible even

to gain more weight than you had before going Ketogenic diet. How then do you overcome that? The first thing to do is to maintain your low-level calorie diet. I told you about habit formation. It is important to develop good habits. Avoid eating processed foods and keep an eye on your carb intake. Once you are able to maintain a good eating habit, you can maintain your weight which you had before you started your Ketogenic diet.

- Loss of Hair: It is possible to experience hair loss when you are making a switch from a Ketogenic diet to other diets or from Ketogenic diet to normal diet. This is the experience that many people have because of the big change from Ketogenic diet to other forms of diet. It is a withdrawal symptom that some people tend to report once making a change from Keto to another form of diet. This experience happens when you are brushing your hair. However, this is temporal as once you make the full adjustment by stopping the Ketogenic diet, it will stop with time.

- Normal Breath: Most Keto dieters experience a lot of bad breath where their breath takes on a fruity smell. This is the because of the ketones that are escaping through their breath. However, when changing from Keto to other forms of diet or normal diet, you are likely to experience good breath.
- A Higher level of Energy: When transitioning from a normal diet to Ketogenic diet, one of the temporal things you will encounter is the lower level of energy that you will experience on your level of endurance. The reason for this is because your body has been used to carbs as a fuel source for many years.

However, as you returned back to normal diet, the experience of higher energy and performance is instant because your body is returning back to what it is used to. This is one of the withdrawal symptoms of Ketogenic diet.

- Adaptable Metabolism: The human body goes through a lot of adaptive changes as you change from one fuel source to another. One of the withdrawal effects that you will notice is the quick adaptability to the new fuel which is the carb that you are used to. But eat carb wisely and watch your calorie intake else you might end up gaining more weight than you had expected.
- Revitalize carb craving: Be careful! One of the withdrawal symptoms that you notice is revitalized carb cravings. You will begin to desire more carbs

than you can imagine. Discipline is your key. If you want to maintain your weight, then you will have to fight your craving for carbs.

Body Reaction to Ketogenic Diet

There are certain things that you need to expect when you are switching from There are certain things that you need to expect when you are switching from either another low carb diet to a Ketogenic diet or from your normal high carb diet to Ketogenic diet. Your body has been used to one type of fuel source – carb. So when a change is made, there are certain reactions to expect. I will mention them here quickly:

- Poor Mental Focus (happens within 2 -3 days of going Keto, it stops with time.)
- Loss of Strength and Endurance Ability.

- Bad Breath (to stop this, drink much salt and water, brush teeth frequently)
- Irregular heartbeats (drink more liquid and salt to stop this)
- Reduced Physical Performance.
- Constipation (mostly for beginners, drink enough water, salt and liquid, and veggies).
- Dehydration (mostly for beginners, drink plenty liquid).
- Muscle Cramps.
- Flu.

CHAPTER SIX

Introduction

We will consider something else for the purposes of effective Ketogenic diet – exercise as a way of furthering your Ketogenic diet. What type of exercise do you need to do that will ensure faster weight loss? We will look at them very briefly.

In the past, there were so many misconceptions about doing a Ketogenic diet and carrying out an exercise. This form of misconception and propaganda has been set in motion by the conjectures flown around on the internet and many research studies. Many of the physicians who fought against being on a Ketogenic diet and engaging in thorough exercise did so because of the insufficient knowledge which they had. Besides, their information was not evidential neither was it factual but on the basis of inchoate knowledge. But as the medical field became agog with information regarding the diet, with many research being birthed on the diet that experts placed participants on a high carb diet, and those on a Ketogenic diet to test the efficacy of their strength during exercise, it was realized that those on the Ketogenic diet did well with an enduring strength.

To begin with, you are closer to the gate of losing weight more effectively when you are on a Ketogenic diet than those who are not on a diet. The reason for this is because when your body is in Ketosis, every bit and ounce of your energy come from fat. In effect, even when your body is in a state of rest, your stored body fat is still being utilized by your body which in turns makes you look slim fit. But with Ketogenic diet, you get better results from your weight loss program when you attach it to some form of exercise. This is very vital; please pay attention. For people who are on a high carb diet, they have to exercise for a long period of time for them to enter into their fat burning point. It may take probably about twenty or more minutes to reach the point of burning fat. On the converse, for people or persons who are on a Ketogenic diet, they are constantly at the state or point of burning fat once ketosis has been attained, hence the potential of your weight loss during a workout is higher. When you decide to work out, you add more lean body muscle that increases the rate of burning energy than when you decide not to work out. The fundamental difference between Keto dieters one on a workout and the other not on a workout program are the ratios of weight loss. While the one on workout loses weight faster, the other one who is not on a workout loses weight at a slower rate compared to the one who is steadily taking in dosages of exercises. It is highly recommended if you want to lose weight faster to adopt an exercise plan that is different from your diet plan. It is essential to know that if you have not been exercising and want to begin one during a Ketogenic diet, it should be done slowly and with time you can increase your workout. Thirty minutes per day of easy cardio will be sufficient. Exercises like – walking, swimming, and resistance training for the purposes of enhancing muscle leanness are good. As your body adapts to regular exercise, you can increase the amount of your workout per day.

Types of Ketogenic Diet for Effective Exercise

As a result of the change in your diet, especially if you are fit and have been exercising regularly, it is possible to feel the absence of glycogen in your muscles. If you are already quite fit and exercise regularly, you may find that the absence of glycogen in your muscles which may sometimes make it difficult for you to be effective in your exercise. Where you find yourself in any of the above-mentioned situations, then the recommendations in this small subhead will be of a pertinent importance to you. For effective exercise tips, it may be possible to attempt a switch from your normal Keto diet to targeted or cyclical Ketogenic diet. We will go ahead to explain these two forms of exercise plan for your Ketogenic diet.

The burning question is, what is a cyclical Ketogenic diet? By definition, a cyclical Ketogenic diet is a standardized procedure for a Ketogenic diet where a person during the week, from Monday to Friday maintains his Ketogenic menu plan strictly but on weekends the amount of carb is increased. In this type of diet plan, the carb load on weekdays is normal while on the weekend; the carb load rate is higher. When you are on a cyclical Ketogenic Diet plan, you will follow a normal diet plan in the course of the week, but at weekends, your diet plan takes a slightly higher amount of carb. When you load carbs this way, it will enable you to store some carb energy for the week so that you can have some level of energy for effective workouts. The only days that you will cut down your carb is Monday to Friday while on Saturday and Sunday, you increase the amount of carb intake. In this diet plan, your first 14 days will be the inducement stage where you essentially stick to a low carb Ketogenic diet plan in order for you to go into full blown ketosis. Once you have achieved ketosis, then you can then follow your cyclical Ketogenic diet plan. However, a different plan might work for you.

The Targeted Ketogenic diet plan. Let us make an attempt at explaining what it means. A targeted Ketogenic diet plan means eating more amount of carbs before workouts. In other words, in this type of diet plan, a person will adopt a low carb diet, mainly adhering to his Ketogenic diet plan every day of the week but when the days for the exercise or workouts comes, an extra gram of carb is consumed before exercise. The purpose for this is to boost your glucose to have more energy for the exercise. One good thing about this diet plan is that it does not stop your body from returning back to ketosis status when you are through with your exercise. However, as a note of advice, I will caution you a little about following a cyclical or target Ketogenic diet plan. Why? It is very easy to begin to use the excuse of these diet plans and start to consume excess carbs. If you do this, it will easily throw you out of ketosis. When on a cyclical or targeted diet plan, it is good to avoid fructose type of food and consume more foods that are glucose or dextrose based. The reason for this is because fructose will likely interrupt your ketosis status. If you decide on any of the above-mentioned types of diet that you will want to adapt to make your workouts and cardio exercise very efficient, you must avoid these list of foods which have very high fructose content, so you do not fall out of ketosis:

1. Carbonated beverage drinks such as soda

2. Pomegranate juice, especially the one that is bottled.

3. Medjool

4. Nectar from mango

5. Carbonated beverage drink such as ginger ale

6. Tamarind Nectar

7. Raisins

8. Applesauce

9. Ketchup

10. Agave

11. Cranberry juice

12. Cherries

13. Persimmons

14. Vinegar

15. Asparagus

16. Dates

It is important to watch out for these types of food when you have decided that you want to undertake a cyclical or targeted Ketogenic diet. Most of the carbonated beverage drinks have very high level of fructose chief among them sodas like coca-cola, Pepsi, mountain dew, etc. these companies use high fructose corn syrup in their products giving it an unlikely high sweetness. Instead of these types of foods, eat foods that are rich in glucose for either of these diets that you have undertaken. Foods like:

- Grains

- Cereal
- Veggies
- Some Nuts and Seeds
- Leguminous foods
- Honey
- Breakfast cereals

General Advise Tips

From the beginning of this book down to the end of it, it is information-packed. We started from the early stage by telling you how the ketone diet came about. However, let me add more value to what your money purchased. I want to give you some general advice tips that will help the course of your weight loss plan.

Planning

Your meals should always be planned ahead of time. The 21-day meal plan outline here is more than silver and gold to help you in your speedy weight loss goals. It is good to think about what you will eat the next day. Always be on the top of your Ketogenic diet game all the time. If during the previous day you have leftovers, make use of them. Do not throw them away. The importance of planning ahead can never be overstated. If during the course of your planning you discovered that there are mistakes in what you are supposed to eat, it is easy to detect them because you have planned ahead. For instance, you can detect if the amount of protein that you are supposed to eat is too high. If the protein is unnecessarily high, it is possible to disturb your ketosis because too much of protein is converted into glucose. Do you see why it is important to plan ahead?

Sleeping and Resting

Sleeping and resting. In recent times, studies have shown that sleep and your appetite are interconnected. This is because your sleep affects the balance of your leptin and ghrelin in the body. Grehlin is a hormone that is produced when a person is hungry, increases your eating appetite. But leptin performs a different function in the body. It is the one that tells the brain that you are full and satisfied so that you don't overeat. Studies have shown that during sleep deprivation leptin level goes down. This decrease in appetite affects your level of satiation. A study was done by doctors who subjected about 12 persons to 2 days of enough sleep and another set of 2 days of sleep deprivation. It was observed during the research that in the two days of sleeplessness, the level of leptin in the body reduced while the level of ghrelin in the body increased. As a result of this, their appetites increased with a resultant effect on their desire for food and calories which equally experienced a tremendous increase. Another research that tested leptin and Grehlin level and body fat percentage, it revealed that the participants in the study that had less than 8 hours sleep per night experienced increased levels of hormonal activity mainly the ghrelin which instigates the feeling of hunger. I will recommend that if you have insomnia, you should avoid eating your dinner shortly before bedtime. Besides that, always ensure that you have a good sleeping schedule and then cut down on the amount of caffeine in your diet. If you do all of these things and nothing still happens, or you find yourself unable to sleep, darken your room at night before bedtime. You can even resort to the use of a natural supplement to help you find rest at night.

Support Group

Now, like should attract like. It is very good to look for a support group that can help you. There are anti-Ketone dieters everywhere that are not in agreement with the Ketogenic dieters. If you walk in their counsel, rejection will be the very thing that you will experience. It is very important for you to look for support groups around you, fellow ketone dieters that will be willing to assist you and encourage you. If they lose pounds of weight, they come and tell you what they have lost. It is a popular knowledge that many ketone dieters record a higher level of success when they are with a group that supports them. When you are with your support group, you can ventilate or express your grievances and difficulties without being put down. So you have to look for a community of people that are mostly ketone dieters who will not find your diet discomforting and will be willing to support you. This group, of course, will know what your goals are, they will encourage you to pursue them. On the basis of their experiences, these people can help you, assist you in attaining your goals and they can answer your questions too. For beginners, it is possible to experience some things that you could not have read in this Ketogenic diet book. Your support group experience will come in handy to help you in such situations.

Reward Scheme

Encourage yourself and give yourself a medallion of reward. As you achieve the goals that you have set for yourself, you need to reward yourself. I must state here that, rewarding yourself doesn’t necessarily mean that you have to eat meals that will endanger your Ketone diet or your Ketosis. You can treat yourself to something nice that doesn't put your Ketogenic diet in danger. You can eat something that is not Ketone inclined but watch it carefully so that you don't put so much effort in your Ketone diet and later it becomes a total and colossal waste. It is ideal to set goals for yourself and when you hit the bar of those goals, give yourself a reward. When you meet the first goal, increase the bar and follow it logically until you smash the next bar. When you do that, reward yourself. If you have to feast on anything during your reward, something like pizza, then ensure it is a low carb. This reward scheme and treating yourself to what you have achieved will keep you highly encouraged. The reward scheme is an encouragement system, built by you to encourage no one but you.

Part 5

CHAPTER SEVEN

Low Carb and High Fat (LCHF)

Ketogenic dieting involves the consumption of low carbohydrate food and more of high fat/moderate protein food, fruits and vegetables like an egg, milk, cheese, butter, oranges, avocados, lettuce, spinach, cabbage, cauliflower, onions, and garlic, etc. More high fat foods are consumed in keto diet plan so that the liver can convert excess fat into Ketones which is then used as the source of energy for the body.

CHAPTER EIGHT

Five Simple Steps to Living the Ketogenic Lifestyle

Sometimes adhering to a strict keto dieting could be as difficult as quitting an addiction. However, to reach ketosis, you will have to cultivate a good diet-discipline habit. Here are five steps that will help you go keto successfully.

i. **Restock Your Foodstuffs:** Restocking your foodstuffs in the kitchen will help you a great deal in kick-starting and maintaining your keto diet program. Restock your kitchen with low carb foodstuffs and clear out all high carb foodstuffs from the kitchen because they could be a source of temptation. Also, stock your kitchen and fridge with other low carb snacks, fruits, and vegetables.

ii. **Monitor Your Carb Intake:** This is as important as the above as calculating and monitoring your carb level will help quicken your journey into ketosis. Inasmuch as you curtail your carb intake, do not consume more than 30 net carbs daily. Consume food that contains more of high fat and protein to enhance the rapid production of ketones. Be sure to check the nutritional label of each foodstuff and snacks you buy to see the carb level.

iii. **Carefully Select Eateries:** To sustain a strict keto diet program, you must choose restaurants and eateries you eat; that is if you are the busy workaholic that has no time to cook. Visit special diet eateries that prepare low carb food and snacks that go with your breakfast, lunch, and dinner keto diets like egg omelet and bacon with a cup of coffee for breakfast, chicken, or fish salad for lunch and some hamburger with broccoli and vegetables for dinner. Just try and avoid eateries that serve high carb food like wheat meals and rice.

iv. **Always Check Your Ketone Level:** As you observe the rules for a strict keto dieting, always remember to check your ketone level using a device called *ketostix*. Checking your ketone level will help you know how fast or slow you are going into ketosis and in curtailing your carb consumption to quicken ketosis. You can check your ketone level through your urine dropped on the ketostix.

v. **Irregular Fasting and Regular Exercise:** Irregular fasting during a keto diet program helps the liver in converting fat into ketones which the brain and body will use as fuel.

Fasting helps reduce the glucose level in the body thereby making way for the brain to get used to fat (ketone) as its source of energy. Also, a regular exercise helps the body in fat-burning and helps the body adapt to using fat as the source of energy in the body.

What to do when you are Eating Out

Embarking on keto dieting requires sacrifice and discipline for the desired result to be achieved. Clearing all high carb foodstuffs and restocking your kitchen is the first step when starting keto dieting. This is to avoid the temptation of consuming high carb food while on a keto diet program.

However, when going out to eat in eateries and restaurants, keto dieters are advised to look out for special diet restaurants. Keto dieters should always go for eateries/restaurants that prepare low-carb/high fat meals so as to avoid the temptation of consuming anti-keto meals as hunger could make you compromise.

Part 6

CHAPTER NINE

The Complete Keto Shopping List

KETO MEAT AND POULTRY

Chicken

Turkey

Beef

Eggs

Bacon

Lamb

KETO FISH AND SEAFOOD

Tuna

Salmon

Smoked Salmon

Halibut

Crab

Shrimp

Anchovy

KETO VEGETABLES

Celery stalks

Chive

Kale

Green beans

Mint leaves

Shallot bulb

Rosemary leaves

Fresh Sprigs thyme

Potatoes

Artichokes

Portobello Mushroom

Cilantro

Dill pickle

Cauliflower

Zucchini

Brussels Sprout

Fresh tomatoes

Scallion

Garlic

Onion.

Leafy greens veggies

Parsley

Spinach

Lettuse

Mushroom

Tarragon leaves

Celery

Broccoli

KETO SPICES

Garlic Powder

Cinnamon powder

Chilli pepper

Salt

Nutmeg

Pumpkin

Italian seasoning

Peppercorn

Curry paste

Black pepper

Tarragon

Paprika

Vinegar

Cayenne pepper

Cumin

Ginger

Oregano

Cumin powder

Pysllium husk powder

Salt

Dried Basil

Jelapeno

Pepper

Tomato Paste

KETO FRUITS

Avocado

Apple

Lemon

Ripe Mango

Kalamata Olive

Carrots

Raspberry

Banana

Strawberries

Cashews

Blueberries

KETO FAT AND OIL

Butter

Olive oil

Coconut oil

Vegetable oil

Curry leaves

KETO SAUCES

Red and Green pesto

Mayonnaise

Worcestershire sauce.

Ketchup

Dijon Mustard

Soy sauce

Coconut cream

Sour cream

Tamarin Soy Sauce

Soybeans sauce

Chili paste

Dijon Mustard

Mint sauce

KETO JUICES

Lemon juice

Lime juice

Mango juices

OTHER FOODS

Bread

Cheese

Goat cheese

Cream cheese

Wheat flour

Feta cheese

Pumpkin puree

Oatmeal flour

Salami

Cheddar

Yogurt

Oat

Cream cheese

Chicken broth/beef broth

Flour

Blue cheese

Whole grain Mustard

Shredded parmesan cheese

Velveeta cheese

Baking powder

Parmesan Cheese

Asiago cheese

Tomato paste

Coconut flour

Milk

Italian balsamic Vinegar

Cocoa powder

KETO SWEETNERS

Coconut milk

Vanilla extract

Stevia extract

Chocolate extract

Non-fat almond milk

Honey

KETO NUTS

Walnuts

Pecans

Pistachios

CHAPTER TEN

The 14 Day Meal Plan

To accelerate your journey to ketosis, trying a strict low carb meal plan will help a great deal. For beginning keto dieters, what to eat and how to plan what to eat is a major challenge that they face. But not to worry, here is a 14 Day keto meal plan and recipes for breakfast, lunch, and dinner to help you attain that desired *ketotic state.*

Week One Meal Plan

Day One

Breakfast: Egg Omelet

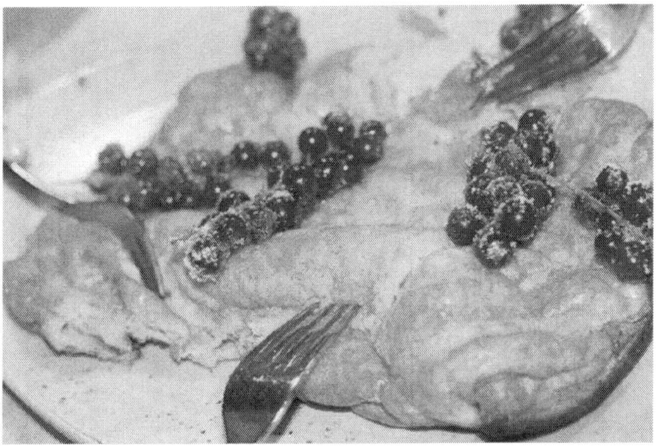

Ingredients:

1. 4 eggs.
2. Butter.
3. 1 minced onion.
4. 1 tsp garlic powder.
5. Salt and ground pepper to taste.

Instruction:

1. Melt butter in a frying pan and watch carefully, so it doesn't burn.
2. Whisk eggs in a bowl. Add onion, garlic, salt, pepper, and mix until fluffy.
3. Pour egg mixture into frying pan containing butter and stir until they become firm.
4. Serve immediately and enjoy.

Lunch: Tuna Cheese Melt

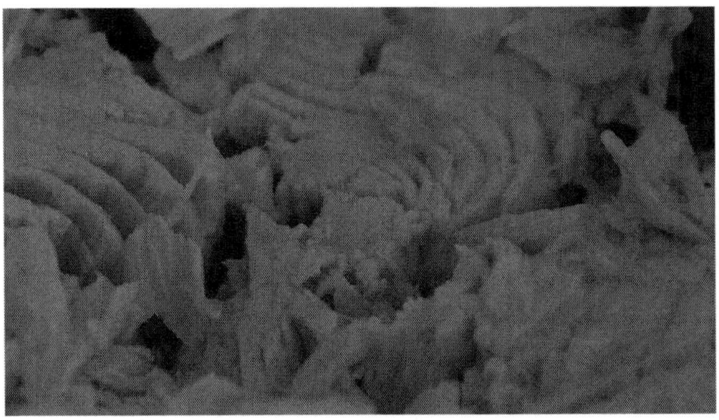

Ingredients:

1. 1 cup of mayonnaise.
2. 4 minced celery stalks.
3. ½ cup chopped dill pickles.
4. 2 cans tuna in olive oil.
5. 1 tsp lemon juice.
6. 1 minced garlic clove.
7. Bread.
8. 4 eggs.
9. leafy greens veggies.
10. Salt and pepper to taste.

Instruction:

1. Preheat oven to 170^{oc}.
2. Mix salad ingredient thoroughly.

3. Place tuna mix into slice bread and apply cheese on top.
4. Add some paprika, cayenne pepper, and garlic spice.
5. Bake for 10-15 minutes.
6. Serve with an olive drizzle over the leafy green.

Dinner: Pesto Chicken with Feta Cheese Spiced using Olives

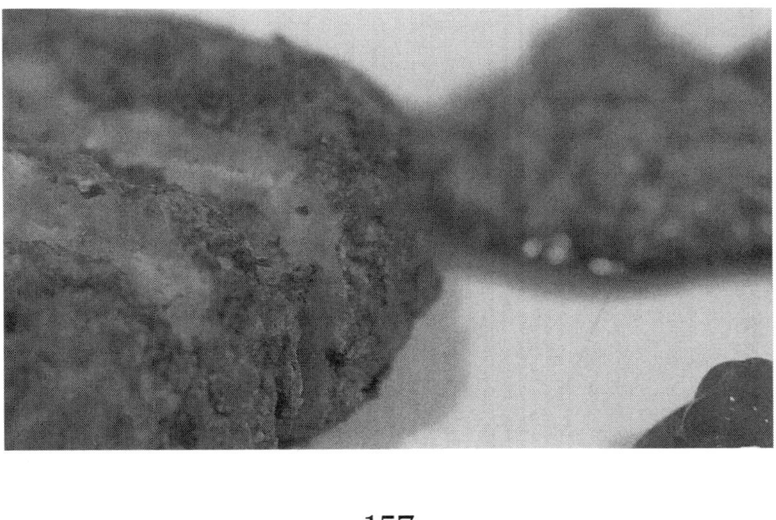

Ingredients:

1. 2 pounds chicken thigh or breast.
2. Red or green pesto.
3. Whipping cream.
4. Pitted olive.
5. Feta cheese.
6. 2 minced garlic cloves.
7. For good taste, use Pepper and salt.
8. Butter for frying.

Instruction:

1. Preheat oven to 200^{oc}.

2. Season cut chicken pieces with salt and pepper then fry in butter till it turns golden brown in colour.
3. Mix pesto and cream in a bowl.
4. Put together fried chicken piece, olives, feta cheese, garlic, and pesto in a baking dish.
5. Bake in oven for 25-30 minutes until it turns brownish in colour.

Day Two

Breakfast

Frittata with Spinach

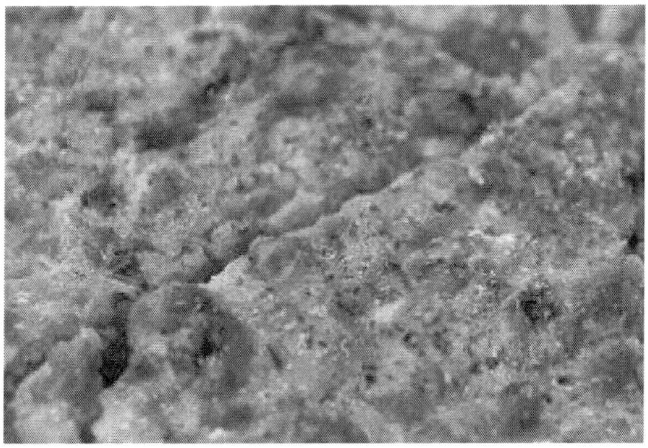

Ingredients:

1. 8 eggs.
2. 1 cup whipping cream.
3. ½ pound fresh minced spinach.
4. 1 pound diced bacon.
5. 1 cup shredded cheese.
6. ½ cup butter for frying.
7. Salt and pepper.

Instruction:

1. Preheat oven to 170°c.
2. Fry the bacon in butter then add the spinach.
3. Mix the eggs and cream together and pour into a baking dish that is greased.
4. Add the bacon, spinach, and cheese on top and place in the middle of the oven.
5. Bake for 25–30 minutes

Lunch: Low-Carbohydrate Meat Pie

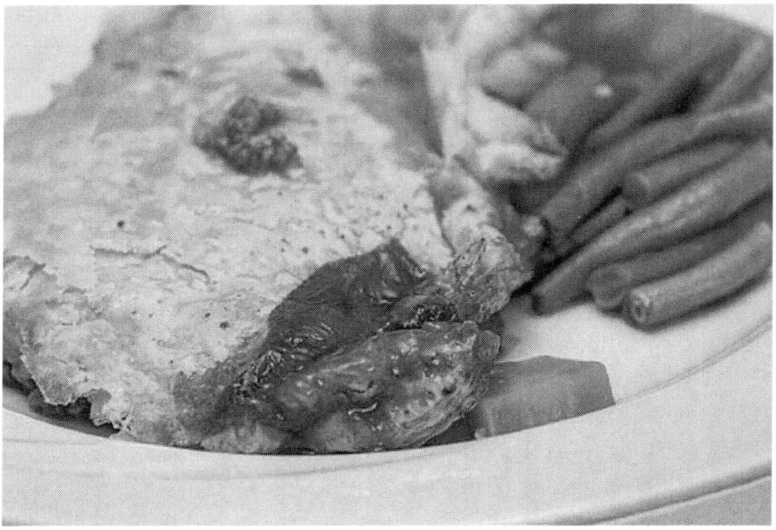

Ingredients:

1. 2 cup of flour.
2. 1 tsp of baking powder.
3. 1 finely minced onion.
4. 2 finely minced garlic clove.
5. ½ cup of butter and olive oil.
6. 1½ pounds shredded beef.
7. Salt and pepper to taste.

8. 2 tbsp dried basil.
9. 5 tbsp tomato paste.
10. ½ cup water.

Instruction:

1. Preheat oven to 180^{oC}.
2. Mix flour, baking powder, butter and egg in a large bowl to form a dough.
3. Over medium heat fry onion and garlic in butter or olive oil until the onion is soft. Then add beef and keep frying.
4. Mix shredded fried beef with olive oil, tomato paste, basil cooking herb, salt, and pepper. Then insert mixture into dough flour mixture for baking.

5. Place dough balls into the well-greased baking pan and bake for 30-40 minutes on medium heat until the pie turns golden brown color.
6. Serve with a fresh green salad as desired.

Dinner: Seared Salmon with lemon

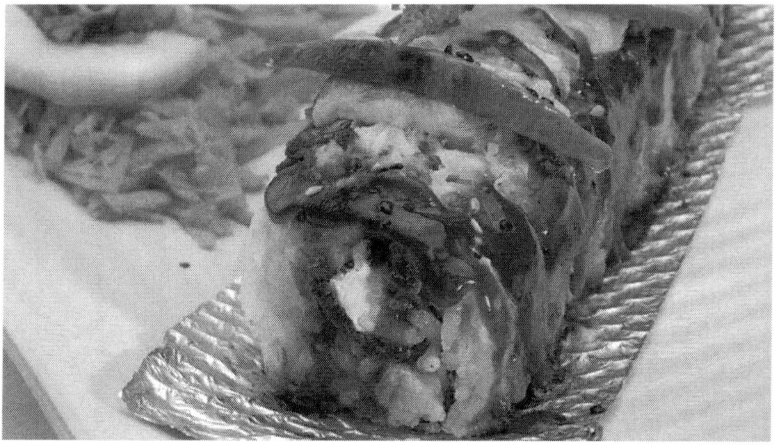

Ingredients:

1. 2 pounds salmon.
2. ½ cup butter.

3. 4 tbsp olive oil.
4. 2 minced garlic cloves.
5. 1 cup lemon juice.
6. 1 big sliced lemon.
7. Salt and ground black pepper for good taste.

Instruction:

1. Preheat oven to 190^{oc}.
2. Place salmon in a greased baking dish and season with salt and pepper.
3. Melt butter and pour some in salmon then slice lemon and place on top. Cover baking dish and bake for 30-40 minutes.

4. Pour remaining butter in a pan over medium heat. Add lemon juice, garlic, salt, pepper, and stir-cook until done.
5. Serve baked salmon on plates and top with lemon butter sauce.

Day Three

Breakfast: Low Carbohydrate Oatmeal

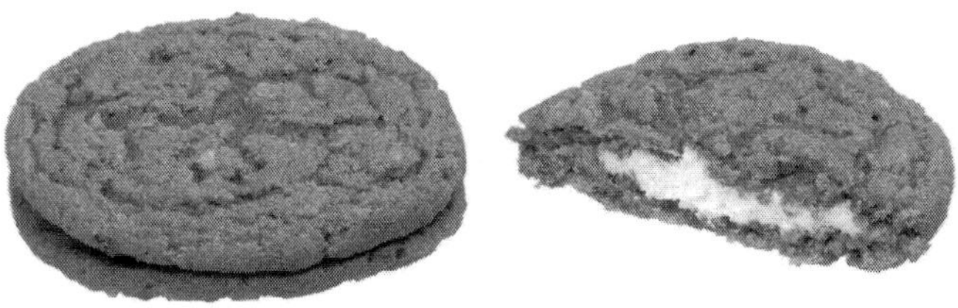

Ingredients:

1. 2 cup oatmeal flour.
2. 1 cup fresh coconut milk.

3. 1 tbsp vanilla extract.
4. 1 tbsp stevia extract or other sweeteners.

Instruction:

1. Mix oatmeal flour in a bowl with little cold water and stir until well mix.
2. Pour hot boiling water to oatmeal and stir until cooked and thick.
3. Add milk, vanilla, Stevie, and stir until well mixed.
4. Serve immediately and enjoy.

Lunch: Salad

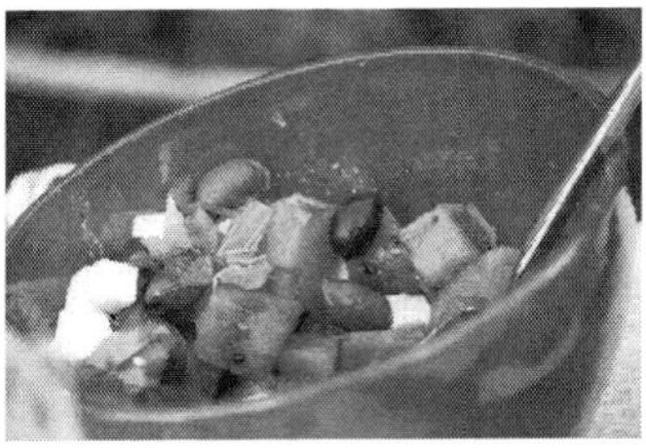

Ingredients:

1. 2 pounds freshly shredded chicken fillet.
2. 1 cup mayonnaise.
3. 2 tbsp olive oil.
4. 2 large avocado.
5. ½ pound leafy green spinach. Finely minced.
6. ½ pound fresh minced lettuce.
7. ½ pound fresh minced cabbage.
8. 1 large finely chopped cucumber.
9. ½ cup finely minced scallion.
10. 4 large fresh minced tomatoes.
11. 2 large diced carrot.

12. Salt and ground pepper to taste.

Instruction:

1. Combine all minced ingredients in a bowl. Add mayonnaise, olive oil, and toss until good mix.
2. Add avocado flesh, carrot, cucumber, salt, pepper, and toss until well mix.
3. Serve in plate and dress with spinach and chicken.

Dinner: Low Carbohydrate Zucchini

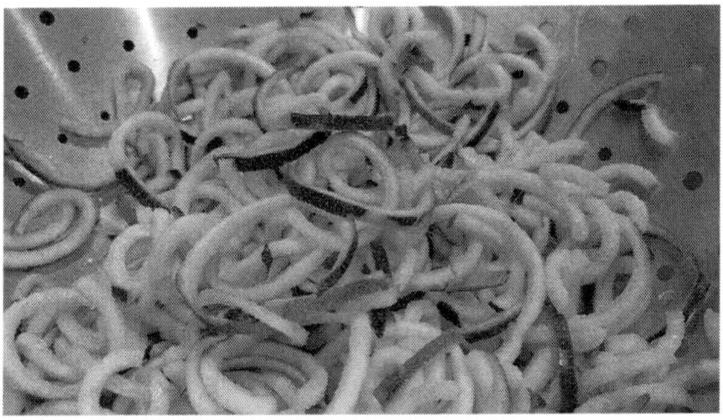

Ingredients:

1. 2 pound fresh zucchini. Trimmed.
2. 1 cup whipping cream.
3. 1 cup grated parmesan cheese.
4. ½ cup mayonnaise.
5. 2 tbsp unsalted butter.
6. 4 egg yolks.
7. 1 pound shredded bacon.
8. 2 tbsp minced parsley.
9. 2 minced garlic cloves.
10. Salt and ground pepper to taste.

Instruction:

1. Melt butter in a pan, add bacon and fry until golden brown.
2. Pour cream into a pot and boil then set aside to cool. Add mayonnaise, salt, pepper and cook for 6-8 minutes.
3. Add zucchini into the heavy creamy mixture and toss until well combined.
4. Serve zucchini in plates and top with cheese, egg, bacon, and parsley. Toss.
5. Enjoy immediately.

Day Four

Breakfast: Coffee Latte

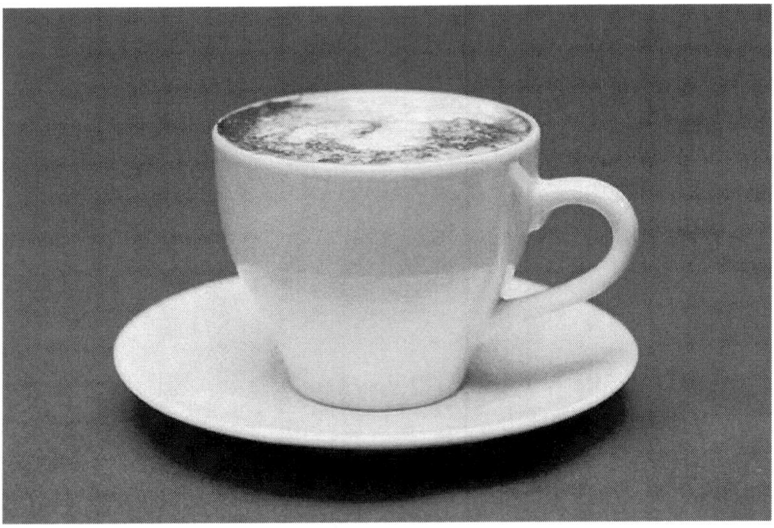

Ingredients:

1. 2 tbsp coffee.
2. 2 eggs.
3. 2 tbsp coconut oil.
4. 1 tsp ginger.
5. ½ tsp vanilla extract.
6. ½ tsp stevia extract.

Instruction:

1. Mix all ingredients in 2 cups of boiling water.
2. Stir and enjoy immediately.

Lunch: Chicken Breast Garnished with Herb Butter

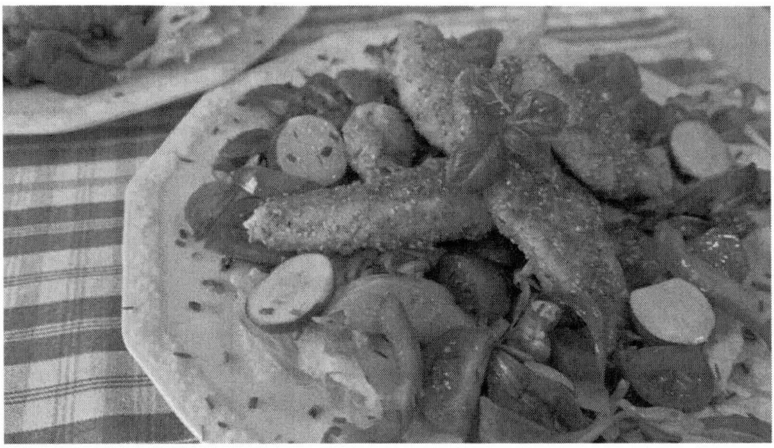

Ingredients:

1. 6 chicken breast.
2. 2 cup unsalted butter.

3. 2 tbsp lemon juice.
4. 4 minced garlic cloves.
5. 4 tbsp minced parsley.
6. ½ pound minced leafy green spinach.
7. Salt and ground black pepper to taste.

Instruction:

1. Melt butter in pan. Season chicken with salt and pepper and fry chicken until golden. Set aside chicken.
2. Pour butter into a bowl. Add garlic, parsley, lemon juice, salt, pepper and toss to form herb butter.

3. Serve chicken over spinach in plates then top with herb butter sauce and enjoy.

Dinner: Low Carbohydrate Beef Casserole

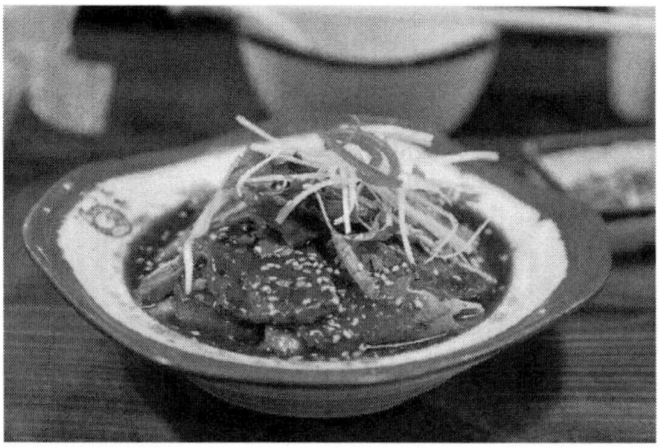

Ingredients:

1. 2 pound shredded beef.
2. 1 cup shredded parmesan cheese
3. 1 cup sour cream.
4. 4 tbsp unsalted butter.
5. 1 can tomato paste.
6. ½ cup minced jalapeno.

7. 1 minced shallot/chive.
8. 1 tbsp ground garlic.
9. 2 tbsp ground paprika.
10. 1 tsp ground cumin.
11. Salt and ground black pepper to taste.

Instruction:

1. Preheat oven to 190^{oc}.
2. Melt butter in a pan and fry beef until golden. Add cumin, paprika, garlic, shallot, tomato and sauté over medium heat for 4 minutes.
3. Pour beef mixture into baking dish; add jalapeno, cheese, and toss well. Bake for 25 minutes.
4. In a small bowl, mix sour cream with chive, salt, pepper, and stir.

5. Serve beef on plates and top with sour cream.

Day Five

Breakfast: Mushroom Omelet

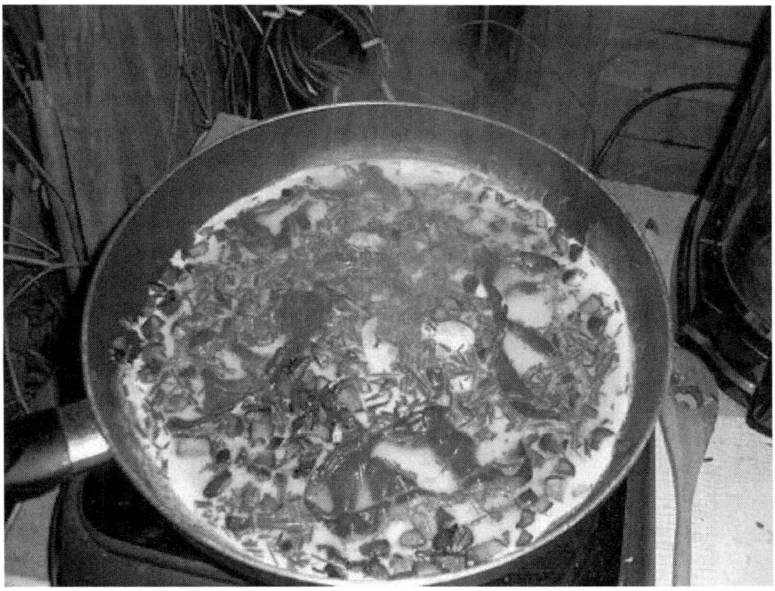

Ingredients:

1. 4 minced mushrooms.

2. 4 eggs.

3. 1 cup shredded cheese.
4. 4 tbsp butter.
5. 1 minced onion.
6. 2 minced garlic cloves.
7. Salt and ground pepper to taste.

Instruction:

1. Break eggs and into a bowl. Add salt and pepper and whisk until well mix.
2. Melt butter in a pan and pour egg mixture into pan. Add mushroom, onion, garlic, cheese and stir until well coated with egg mixture.
3. Allow cooking over moderate heat for 6 minutes (3 minutes each side) until omelet becomes firm and golden all over.
4. Serve immediately and enjoy.

Lunch: Avocado-Bacon and Goat-Cheese Salad

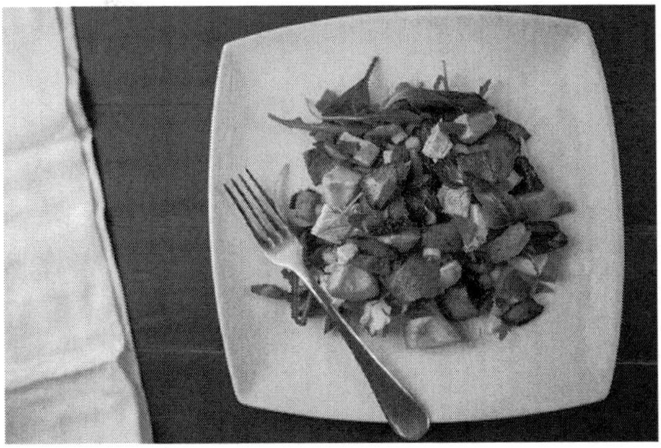

Ingredients:

1. 2 pounds bacon.
2. 4 avocados.
3. 2 cup goat cheese.
4. 1 cup mayonnaise.
5. ½ cup olive oil.
6. 4 tbsp whipping cream.
7. ½ cup lemon juice.

8. 2 pounds fresh minced lettuce.
9. 1 minced shallot.
10. Salt and ground pepper to taste.

Instruction:

1. Preheat oven to 190^{oc}.
2. Melt oil in a pan and fry bacon until light-golden.
3. Place minced lettuce in a bowl. Divide avocados, fetch creamy flesh and put on lettuce.
4. Melt cheese in pan and pour into lettuce. Add bacon and toss.
5. Add mayonnaise, lemon juice, olive oil, whipping cream, salt, pepper and toss until well combined.

6. Serve immediately and enjoy.

Dinner: Brussels Sprouts and Hamburger Gratin

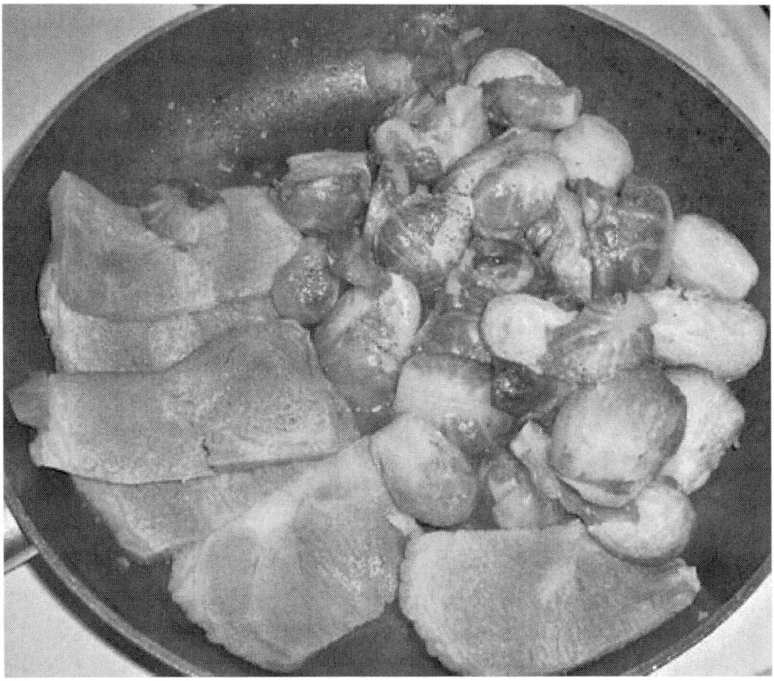

Ingredients:

1. 2 pounds finely diced Brussels sprout.
2. 2 pounds ground beef.

3. 2 cup shredded parmesan cheese.
4. ½ cup unsalted butter.
5. 4 tbsp sour cream.
6. 1 tbsp cumin powder.
7. 6 sprigs minced parsley.
8. Salt and pepper to taste.

Instruction:

1. Preheat oven to 200^{oc}.
2. Melt butter in a pan. Add Brussels sprout and fry until wilt. Season with sour cream and set aside.
3. Season beef with salt and pepper and fry until golden. Add Brussels sprout, cheese, cumin, parsley and stir until well combined.

4. Pour into baking dish and bake in the reheated oven until done.
5. Serve immediately and enjoy.

Day Six

Breakfast: Breakfast Tapas

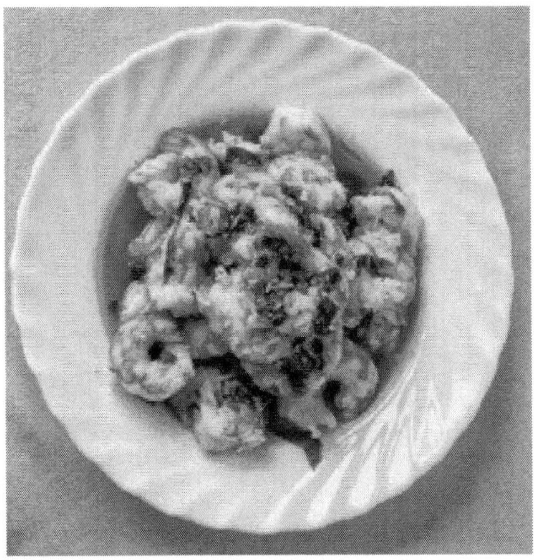

Ingredients:

1. 1 cup shredded cheddar cheese.

2. ½ cup mayonnaise.
3. 2 tbsp lemon juice.
4. 1 pound cold cut bacon.
5. 3 tbsp minced basil.
6. 4 avocados.
7. 2 diced cucumber.
8. 1 cup chopped walnuts.
9. Salt and ground black pepper for a nice taste.

Instruction:

1. Melt cheese in a pan and pour into a bowl. Add mayonnaise, lemon juice, salt, pepper and mix until well combined.
2. Divide avocados and add flesh to cheese mixture. Add bacon, walnut, cucumber and mix until well combined.

3. Serve immediately and enjoy.

Lunch: Pancakes with Spicy Cream-Cheese Topping

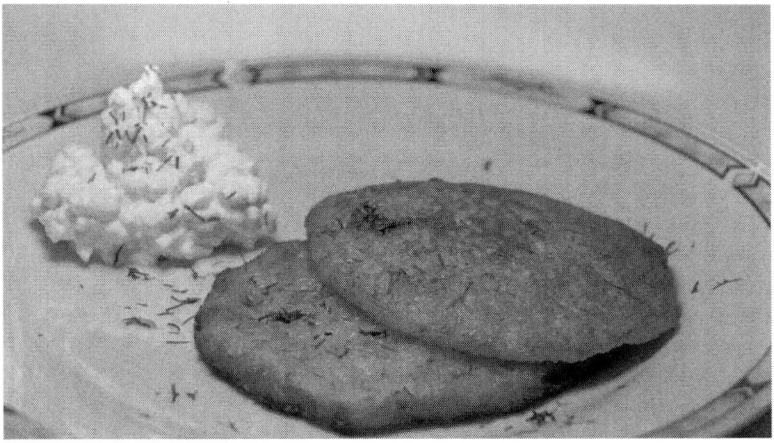

Ingredients:

1. 4 cup white flour.
2. 6 eggs.
3. 1 cup milk.
4. 1 cup cream cheese.

5. 1 cup coconut oil.
6. 4 tbsp basil.
7. 1 tbsp garlic powder.
8. Salt and ground black pepper to taste.

Instruction:

1. Place flour, milk, egg, salt, pepper in a bowl. Mix until smooth and thick to form pancake batter. Shape into small square or ball batter and set aside for frying.
2. Heat oil in pan and fry pancake batter until golden.
3. Pour cream cheese in a bowl. Add oil, basil, garlic, salt, pepper and blend to form cream cheese pesto.

4. Serve pancakes in plates and top with cream cheese pesto.

Dinner: Chops Marinated in Pesto

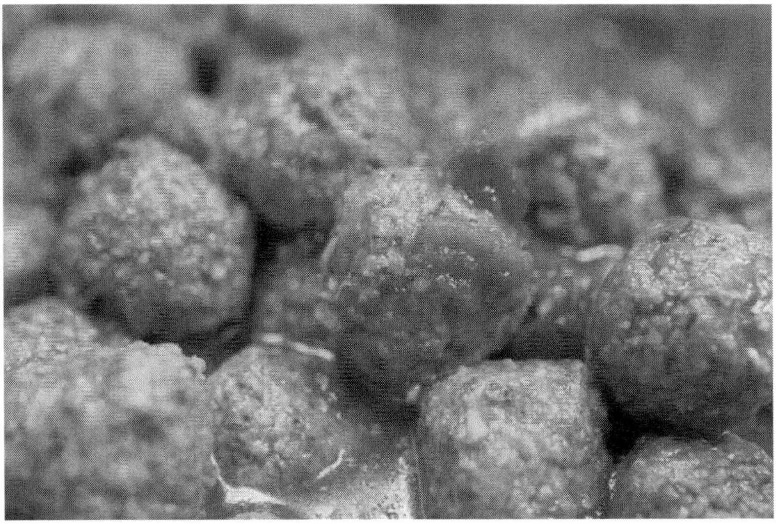

Ingredients:

1. 6 bacon chops.
2. 3 tbsp butter.
3. ½ cup mayonnaise.
4. ½ cup parmesan cheese.

5. 2 tbsp minced basil.
6. 2 tbsp minced parsley.
7. 1 tbsp garlic powder.
8. Salt and ground black pepper to taste.

Instruction:

1. Melt butter in a pan. Add cheese, basil, parsley, garlic, salt, pepper and cook until well combined and thick to form a pesto.
2. Add mayonnaise to pesto and blend.
3. Serve bacon chops and top with pesto sauce.
4.

Day Seven

Breakfast: Bacon Lettuce and Tomato Salad

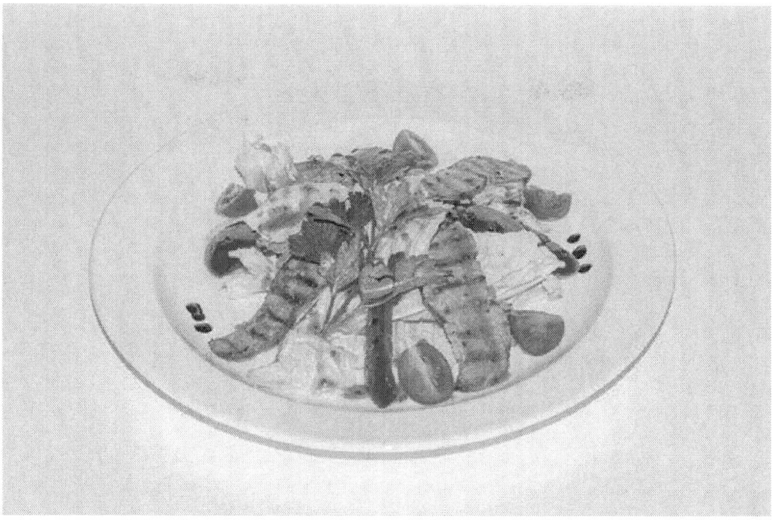

Ingredients:

1. 5 large shredded bacon.
2. 2 heads of fresh lettuce. Sliced.
3. 4 large tomatoes. Sliced.
4. 1 cup of milk.
5. ½ cup of mayonnaise.
6. 1 teaspoon of garlic powder.
7. 1 teaspoon of black pepper powder.

8. Salt to taste.

Instruction:

1. Cook shredded bacon over medium heat until it turns brownish.
2. Place milk, mayonnaise, garlic and pepper in a blender and blend until smooth.
3. Place tomatoes, lettuce, and bacon in a bowl.
4. Pour blended content into the bowl containing tomatoes, lettuce, and bacon and blend together.
5. Serve immediately as desired.

Lunch: Egg Wraps with Shrimp Salad

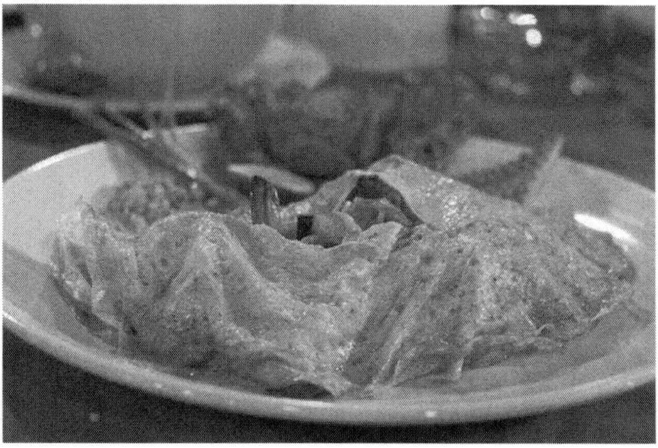

Ingredients:

1. 2 pounds cooked shrimp.
2. 5 eggs.
3. 3 avocados.
4. 1 cup mayonnaise.
5. ½ cup butter.
6. 1 minced lettuce head.
7. 1 diced apple.
8. 2 tbsp lime juice.

9. ½ cup minced parsley.
10. 2 minced garlic cloves.
11. 1 tbsp minced red chili pepper.
12. Salt and ground black pepper to taste.

Instruction:

1. Melt butter in a pan and whisk eggs with salt and pepper in a bowl to prepare egg wraps.
2. Pour whisk eggs into the pan with butter and fry over medium heat until light-golden and firm. Cover and set aside.
3. Place minced lettuce in a bowl. Divide avocados and fetch creamy flesh into bowl with lettuce.

4. Add cooked shrimp, mayonnaise, lemon juice. Apple, parsley, garlic, salt pepper and toss until well combined.
5. Serve egg wrap on plates and top with shrimp salad.

Dinner: Bacon Wrapped Meatloaf

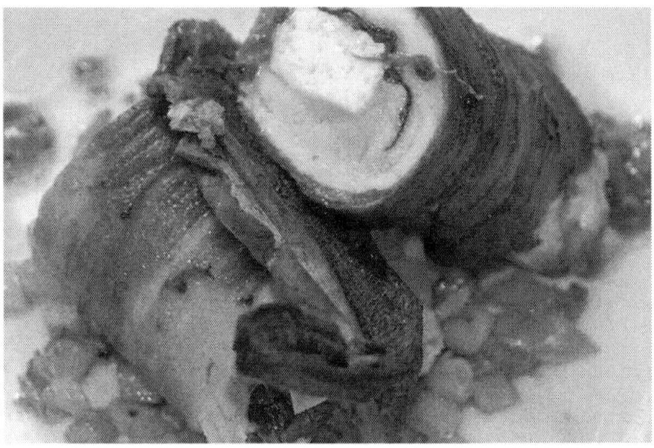

Ingredients:

1. 2 pound shredded bacon.
2. 1 pound ground beef.

3. 2 eggs
4. 4 tbsp unsalted butter.
5. ½ cup shredded cheese.
6. ½ whipping cream.
7. 2 tbsp minced oregano.
8. 4 minced garlic cloves.
9. 1 large minced onion.
10. Salt and ground black pepper powder to taste.

Instruction:

1. Preheat oven to 200^{oc}.
2. Melt butter in a pan and sauté onion.

3. Place ground beef in a bowl. Add egg, butter, cheese, oregano, garlic, salt, pepper and blend until well combined.
4. Roll mixture into small loaf shape and place on a tray. Carefully insert loaf into bacon and put into baking dish.
5. Bake bacon meatloaf for 40 until light-golden. Mix cream with oil, salt, and pepper.
6. Serve meatloaf with cream sauce.

Part 7

CHAPTER ELEVEN

Week Two Meal Plan

Day Eight

Breakfast: Ham Sandwich

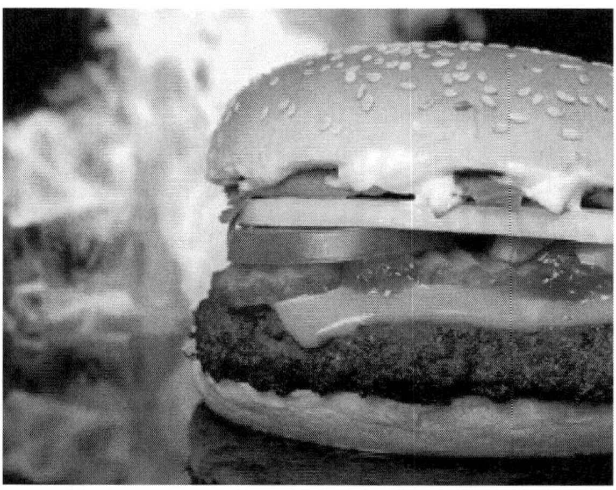

Ingredients:

1. 1 pound ham.
2. 6 eggs.
3. 4 tbsp olive oil.
4. ½ cup shredded cheddar cheese.
5. 1 tbsp Worcestershire sauce.
6. 1 tsp garlic powder
7. Salt and ground black pepper to taste.

Instruction:

1. Whisk eggs in a bowl. Add garlic, salt, pepper and whisk until well combined.
2. Heat oil in a pan and fry eggs until light-golden on both sides. Cover and set aside.
3. Fry ham in oil until golden.

4. Serve ham on plates with cuts of fried eggs. Top with cheese and sprinkle Worcestershire sauce on top.

Lunch: Fish with Curry and Coconut Cream

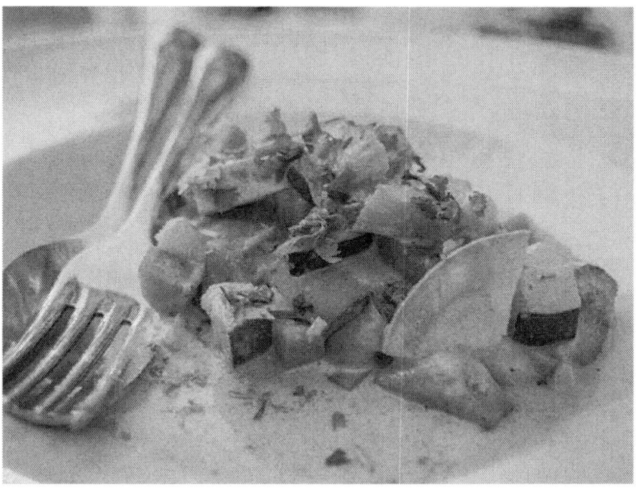

Ingredients:

1. 2 pounds fresh halibut.
2. 1 can coconut cream.
3. 2 tbsp red curry paste.

4. 2 tbsp oil.
5. 2 tbsp butter.
6. 1 head minced broccoli.
7. 4 sprig minced curry leaves.
8. 4 tbsp minced basil.
9. Salt and ground black pepper to have a nice taste.

Instruction:

1. Preheat oven to 190^{oc}.
2. Boil broccoli in salted water until wilt. Drain and cover.
3. Grease baking dish with oil and pour fish in the dish. Add butter, coconut cream, curry

paste/leaves, basil salt, pepper and mix well with fish until well marinated.

4. Bake mixture in preheated oven for 25 minutes until done.
5. Serve halibut with broccoli and enjoy.

Dinner: Hamburger Patties with Creamy Tomato Sauce and Fried Cabbage

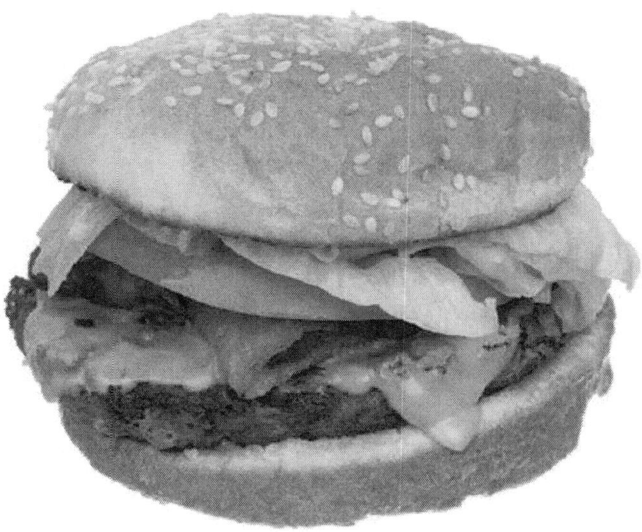

Ingredients:

1. 2 pounds ground beef.
2. 2 cup heavy whipping cream.
3. ½ cup unsalted butter.
4. 1 cup parmesan cheese.
5. 1 small can tomato paste.
6. ½ cup minced parsley.
7. 4 minced garlic cloves.
8. 2 pounds freshly minced cabbage.
9. Salt and ground black pepper to taste.

Instruction:

1. Place ground beef in a bowl. Add some butter, cheese, eggs, olive oil, salt, pepper and blend

until well combined and thick and form into small hamburger patties.

2. Melt butter and oil in a pan and fry over medium heat until patties turn light-golden.
3. Pour tomato paste and whipping cream into the pan with oil and sauté. Reduce heat add fried hamburger patties and simmer to marinate with tomato paste mixture.
4. Melt remaining butter in a pan and sauté minced cabbage, garlic, and parsley until wilt. Add salt and pepper and toss.
5. Serve hamburger and top with fried cabbage.

Day Nine

Breakfast: Coffee

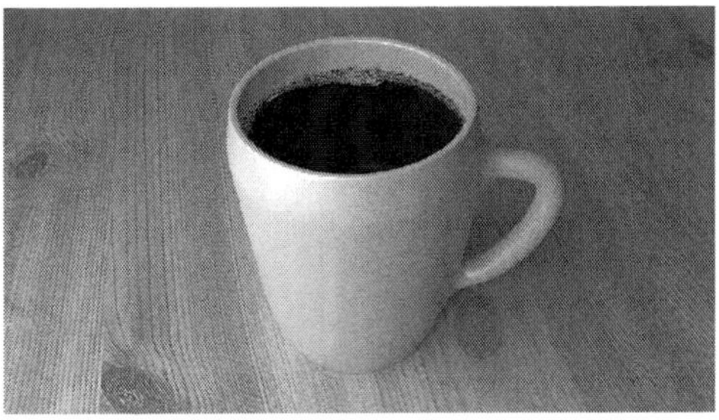

Ingredients:

1. 3 tbsp fresh coffee.
2. 1 tbsp unsalted butter.
3. 1 tbsp coconut oil.
4. 1 tsp stevia extract.

Instruction:

1. Place all ingredients in a cup and full cup with hot boiling water. Stir until good mix.
2. Enjoy immediately

Lunch

Chicken Stroganoff

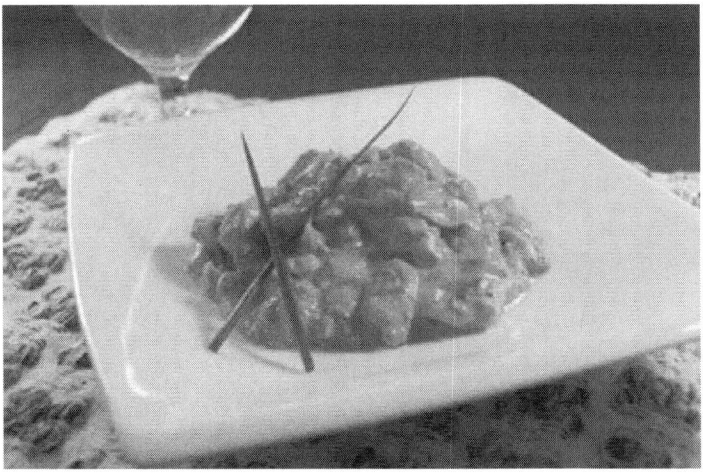

Ingredients:

1. 2 pounds shredded chicken.
2. 1 cup blue cheese.
3. 4 tbsp olive oil.
4. 4 tbsp unsalted butter.
5. 2 cup sour cream.
6. 1 pound minced mushroom.

7. 1 pound zucchini.
8. 1 large minced onion.
9. 2 minced garlic cloves.
10. 2 tbsp oregano.
11. 2b tbsp dried thyme.
12. Salt and ground black pepper to taste.

Instruction:

1. Melt butter in a pan and fry the minced onion until wilt. Add shredded chicken and fry until light- golden.
2. Add minced mushroom and sauté until mushroom wilt.

3. Add sour cream, cheese, thyme, salt, pepper. Stir until well combined then simmer for 12 minutes. Cover and set aside.
4. Cut zucchini then use a spiralizer to trim into zoodles.
5. Heat oil in a pan and add oregano, salt, pepper to make pesto sauce. Add zucchini and sauté until it marinates well.
6. Serve chicken and top with zucchini pesto.

Dinner

Salmon Tandoori Sauced with Cucumber

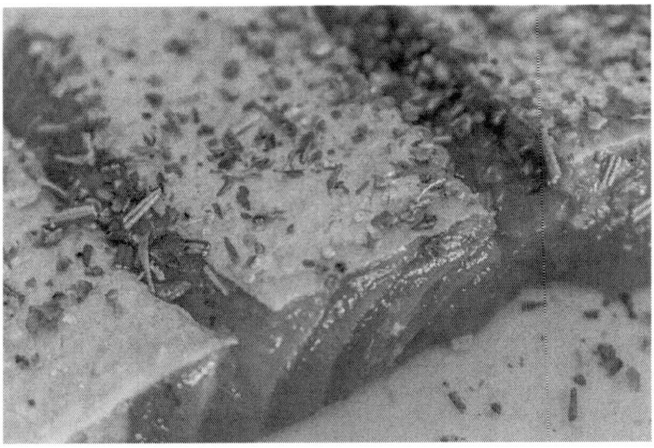

Ingredients:

1. 2 pounds fresh salmon.
2. 1 large dice cucumber.
3. 1 head minced lettuce.
4. 3 avocados.
5. 2 minced onion.
6. 4 tbsp coconut oil.
7. 2 cups sour cream.
8. 4 tbsp lime juice.

9. 1 tbsp garlic powder.
10. Salt and ground pepper to taste.

Instruction:

1. Preheat oven to 180^{oc}.
2. Season salmon with salt, pepper, garlic and fry in oil until light-golden. Cover and set aside.
3. Place cucumber in a bowl, add sour cream, lime juice, garlic salt, pepper and toss well. Cover and set aside.
4. Place minced lettuce in a bowl. Add lime juice, onion, avocado flesh, pepper and toss well.
5. Serve salmon over lettuce salad on plates and top with cucumber sauce.

Day Ten

Breakfast

Coconut Porridge

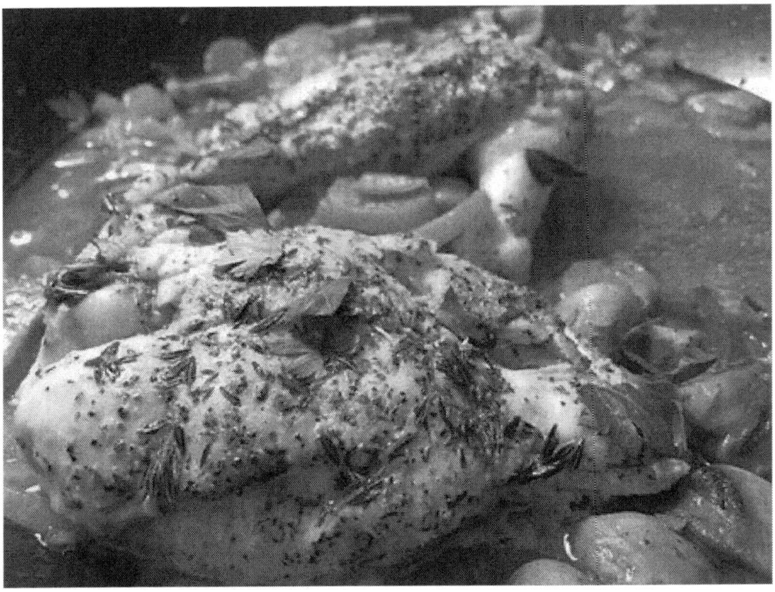

Ingredients:

1. ½ cup coconut flour.
2. ½ cup coconut cream.
3. 2 large eggs.

4. 2 tbsp unsalted butter
5. ½ tsp psyllium husk powder.
6. A pinch of salt.

Instruction:

1. Whisk eggs in a bowl. Add butter, coconut flour, psyllium husk powder, salt and stir until well combined.
2. Pour mixture into a pan over medium heat and stir-cook until thick.
3. Serve in cups with coconut cream and enjoy.

Lunch

Chili Salmon covered with Spinach

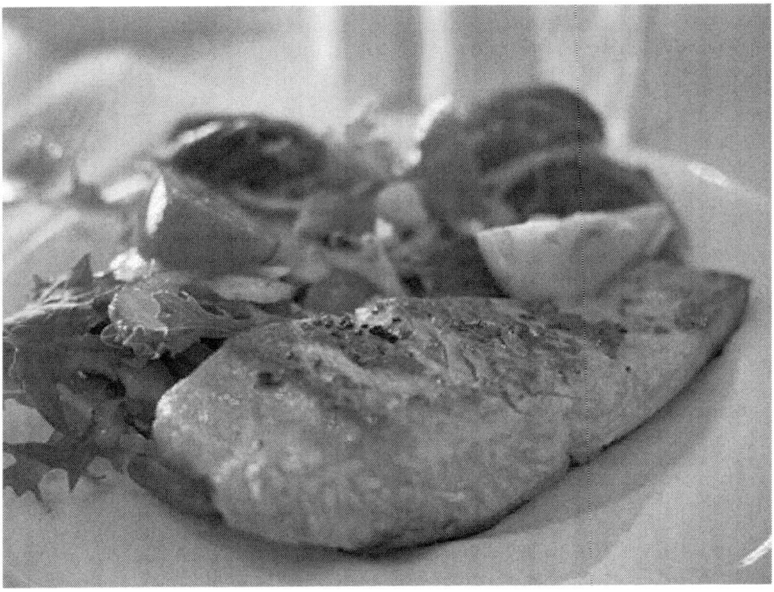

Ingredients:

1. 2 pounds fresh salmon fillets.
2. 1 pound fresh minced spinach.
3. 2 tbsp chili paste.
4. 4 tbsp butter.
5. 4 tbsp mayonnaise.
6. ½ shredded parmesan cheese.

7. 2 tbsp dried basil.
8. Salt and ground pepper to taste.

Instruction:

1. Preheat oven to 190^{oc}.
2. Season salmon with salt, pepper, and place in a greased baking dish.
3. Pour mayonnaise in a bowl and add cheese, chili paste, basil. Stir until well mix and pour into baking dish with salmon.
4. Bake for 20 minutes until salmon is well marinated and done.
5. Melt some butter in pan. Add spinach, salt, pepper and sauté until spinach wilt.
6. Serve salmon over spinach and enjoy.

Dinner

Garlic Chicken

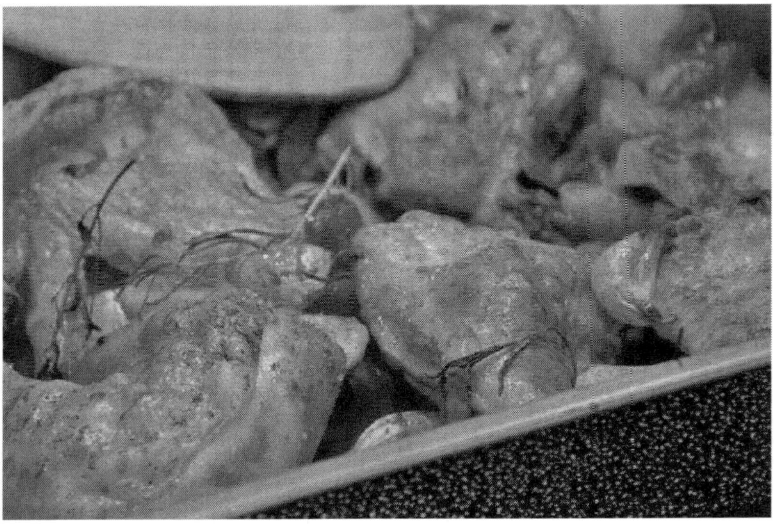

Ingredients:

1. 4 pounds cooked chicken thighs.
2. 6 minced garlic cloves.
3. 2 tbsp garlic powder.
4. 4 tbsp minced parsley.

5. ½ cup olive oil.
6. 5 tbsp butter.
7. 4 tbsp lime juice.
8. Salt and ground black pepper to taste.

Instruction:

1. Preheat oven to 240^{oc}.
2. Place cooked chicken in a greased baking dish. Add melted butter, lime juice, garlic cloves/powder, parsley and stir for the chicken to marinate.
3. Bake in preheated oven for 40 minutes until golden.
4. Serve immediately and enjoy.

Day Eleven

Breakfast

Egg Muffins

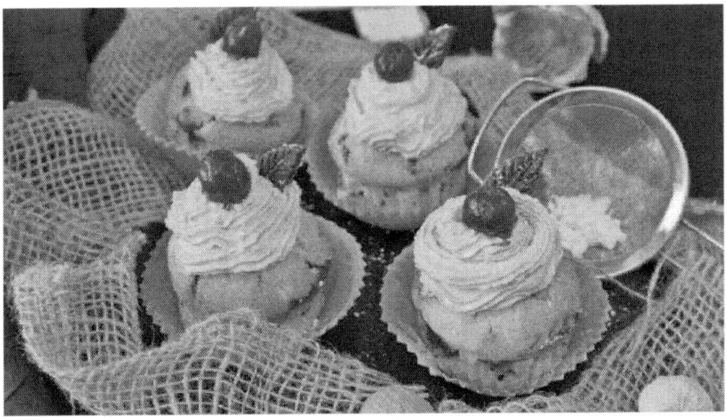

Ingredients:

1. 10 large eggs.
2. 1 cup shredded cheese.
3. 2 tbsp red pesto.
4. 6 tbsp diced salami.
5. 2 tbsp dried chive.
6. 2 finely minced scallion.

7. Salt and ground black pepper to taste.

Instruction:

1. Preheat oven to 180^{oc}.
2. Whisk egg with pesto in a bowl. Add cheese, scallion, chives, salt, pepper and stir until well combined.
3. Pour mixture into muffins and insert diced salami. Place muffins in baking dish.
4. Bake for 20 minutes until firm and golden.
5. Serve immediately and enjoy.

Lunch

Cauliflower Soup with Crumbled Bacon

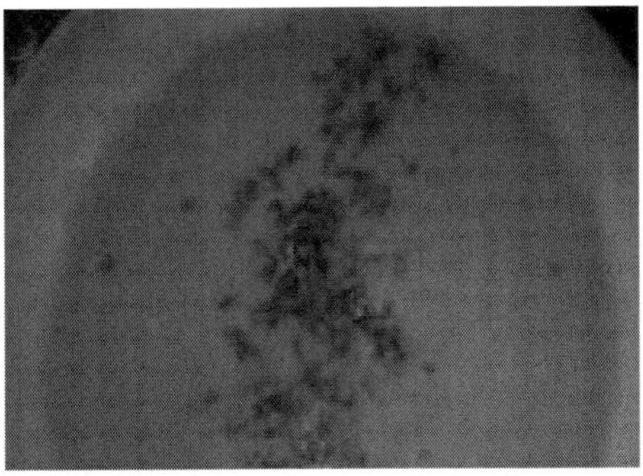

Ingredients:

1. 2 pounds shredded bacon.
2. 1 pound finely minced cauliflower.
3. 1½ cup cream cheese.
4. ½ cup unsalted butter.
5. 2 cup chicken or beef broth.
6. 2 tbsp Dijon mustard.
7. ½ cup shredded pecan nuts.
8. 2 tbsp paprika powder.
9. 1 tbsp garlic powder.

10. Salt and ground pepper to taste.

Instruction:

1. Melt butter in pan. Add crumbled bacon and fry until light-golden. Remove bacon from oil and set aside.
2. Add minced cauliflower, garlic, paprika, pecan nuts, salt, pepper and sauté until cauliflower wilt.
3. Add chicken broth to cauliflower and bring to boil. Add cream cheese, butter, mustard and cook over medium heat until done.
4. Serve crumbled bacon on plates and top with cauliflower soup.

Dinner

Pork Chops with Blue-Cheese Sauce

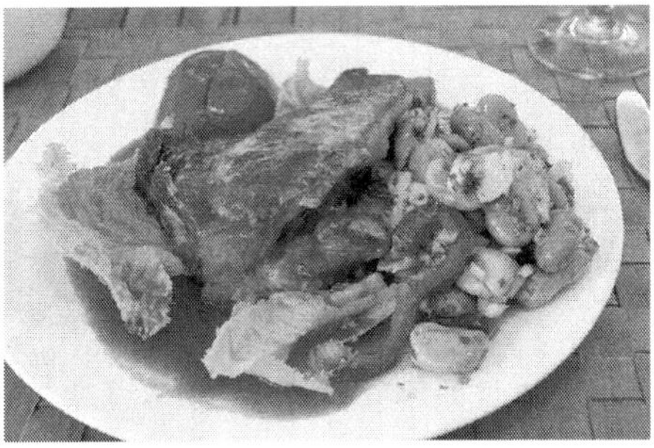

Ingredients:

1. 6 large pork chops.
2. 1½ cup blue cheese.
3. 1 cup sour cream.
4. 4 tbsp butter.
5. 1 cup fresh diced green beans.
6. 1 tbsp dried basil.
7. 2 minced garlic cloves.
8. Salt and ground black pepper to taste.

Instruction:

1. Melt butter in pan. Add pork chops and season with salt, pepper and fry until golden. Cover and set aside.
2. Add green beans to butter and sauté the cover and set aside.
3. Melt cheese over medium heat in a pan. Add sour cream, stir and let it cook for 10 minutes.
4. Reduce heat and add basil, garlic, a little salt, pepper; stir and simmer until thick.
5. Serve pork chops with green beans and top with blue cheese sauce.

Day Twelve

Breakfast

Scrambled Eggs with Cheese

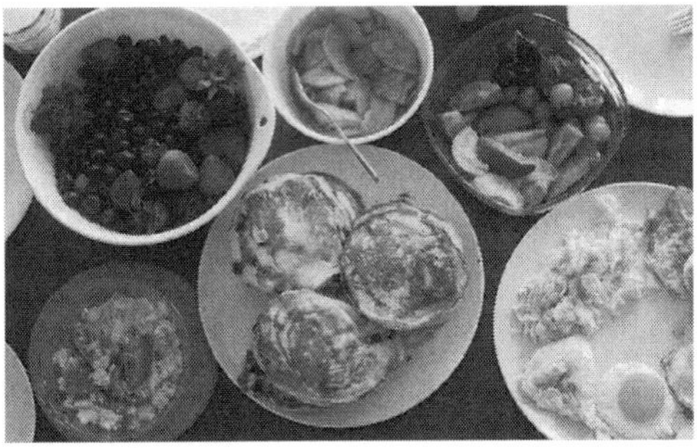

Ingredients:

1. 8 large eggs.
2. 1 pound shredded bacon.
3. 1½ cup feta cheese.
4. 4 tbsp olive oil.
5. 2 large diced scallions.
6. 4 minced garlic cloves.
7. ½ cup finely minced parsley.
8. Salt and ground black pepper to taste.

Instruction:

1. Whisk eggs, parsley, garlic, salt and pepper in a bowl.
2. Heat oil in a pan. Add bacon, scallions and fry until golden.
3. Pour whisk egg in a pan with bacon. Add cheese, stir and sauté for minutes until firm.
4. Serve immediately and enjoy.

Lunch

Tortilla with Crushed Beef and Salsa

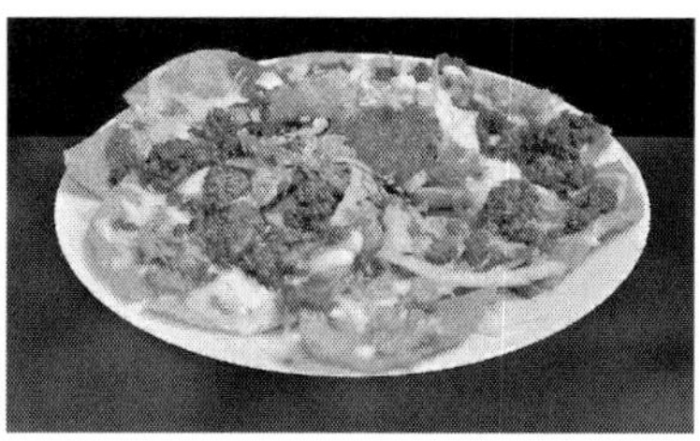

Ingredients:

1. 2 pounds ground beef.
2. 2 cup cream cheese.
3. 1 cup shredded cheese.
4. ½ cup olive oil.
5. 8 eggs.
6. 4 avocados.
7. ½ cup lime juice.
8. 1 pounds leafy greens.
9. ½ cup minced cilantro.
10. 4 finely minced tomatoes.
11. 1 tsp cumin/chili/paprika/garlic powder.
12. 2 tbsp ground psyllium husk powder.
13. 4 tbsp coconut flour.
14. Salt and ground black pepper to taste.

Instruction:

1. Preheat oven to 200^{oc}.
2. Place egg, cream cheese, salt and pepper and whisk until smooth.
3. Add coconut flour, psyllium husk powder and whisk until batter turns thick.
4. Place parchment paper on baking sheet and make thin circles with batter and bake in preheated oven until light-golden. Cover and set aside fried tortillas.
5. Heat oil in a pan and sauté ground beef for 12 minutes. Add some water, salt, pepper and simmer until water drains. Summer leafy greens in hot salty water.

6. Divide avocados and fetch flesh into a bowl. Add lime juice, olive oil, cumin, chili, paprika, garlic, tomatoes, 4 tbsp cilantro, salt, pepper and toss until well combined to for salsa.
7. Serve fried tortillas with ground beef over salsa sauce and leafy greens.

Dinner:

Fish Casserole spiced Mushroom and Mustard

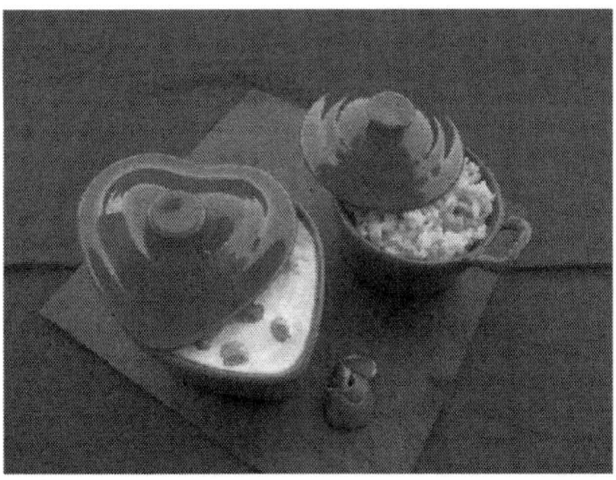

Ingredients:

1. 2 pounds fresh salmon fillets.
2. 1 pound mushroom.
3. 4 tbsp Dijon mustard.
4. 1 pound broccoli.
5. ½ cup unsalted butter.
6. 1 cup shredded cheese.
7. 1 cup heavy whipping cream.
8. 2 tbsp dried basil.
9. 1½ tbsp garlic powder.
10. Salt and ground black pepper to taste.

Instruction:

1. Preheat oven to 180^{oc}.

2. Melt butter in a pan and fry mushroom until wilt. Add salt, pepper, parsley, heavy cream, mustard and simmer for 10 minutes.
3. Place salmon in a greased baking dish and season with salt and pepper. Add creamed mushroom and bake in preheated oven for 25 minutes until fish is done.
4. Cut broccoli into florets and boil in lightly salted water. Drain and add butter, salt, pepper, and toss.
5. Serve baked fish with broccoli and enjoy.

Day Thirteen Breakfast: Eggs and Bacon

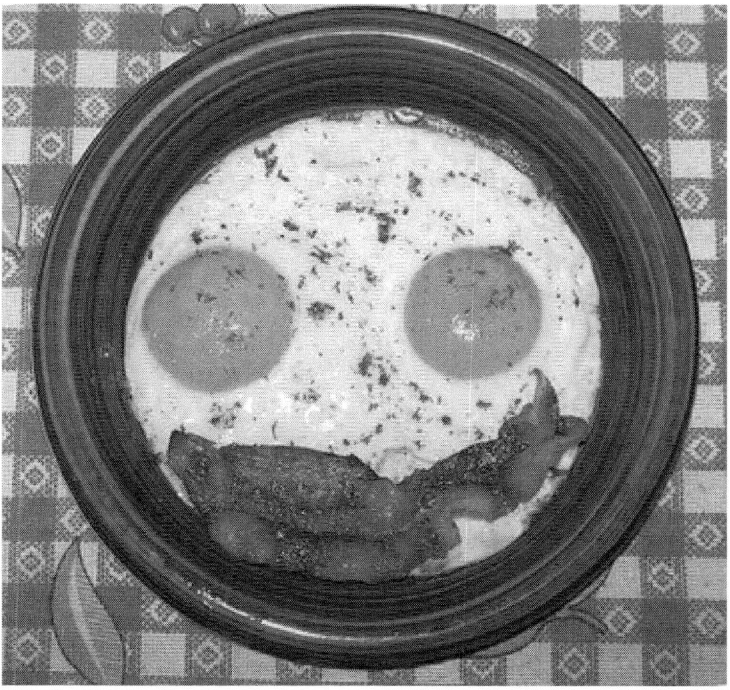

Ingredients:

1. 10 eggs.
2. 2 pounds shredded bacon.
3. 4 tbsp olive oil.
4. 2 finely minced scallions.
5. 2 large minced tomatoes.

6. 4 tbsp minced parsley.
7. 1 tbsp garlic powder.
8. Salt and ground pepper to taste.

Instruction:

1. Heat oil in a pan and fry bacon until golden. Cover and set aside.
2. Whisk eggs in a bowl. Add scallions, tomato, parsley, garlic, salt, pepper and fry in a pan with oil until golden.
3. Serve bacon on plates and top with fried eggs.

Lunch

Salmon with Pesto and Spinach

Ingredients:

1. 2 pounds fresh salmon fillets.
2. 1 cup parmesan cheese.
3. ½ cup mayonnaise.
4. 6 tbsp olive oil.
5. 1 pound fresh minced spinach.
6. 2 tbsp dried basil.
7. 1 tsp garlic powder.
8. 1 sachet tomato paste.
9. Salt and ground black pepper to taste.

Instruction:

1. Preheat oven to 190^{oc}.
2. Season salmon fillets with salt and pepper and place in a greased baking dish.

3. Whisk cheese and mayonnaise in a bowl. Add oil, basil, garlic, tomato paste, salt, pepper and stir until well mix.
4. Pour in a baking dish with salmon and toss. Bake in preheated oven for 20 minutes until salmon is done and golden.
5. Season spinach with little salt and pepper and sauté minced spinach in a pan with oil until wilt.
6. Serve salmon with spinach and enjoy.

Dinner

Beef Steak with Béarnaise Sauce

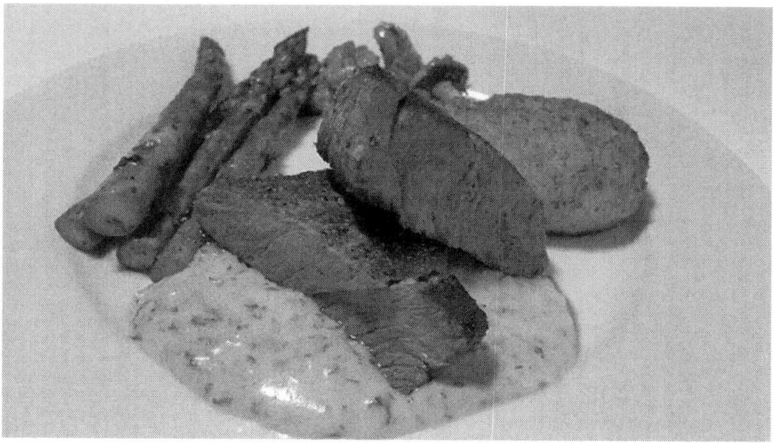

Ingredients:

1. 8 fresh beef steak.
2. 8 egg yolks.
3. 4 tbsp finely minced tarragon.
4. 1 cup unsalted butter.
5. 1 pound finely minced lettuce.
6. 4 minced tomatoes.
7. 1 tbsp garlic powder.
8. 2 tbsp onion powder.

9. 4 tbsp vinegar.
10. Salt and ground black pepper to taste.

Instruction:

1. Melt butter in a hot pan.
2. Whisk egg yolks in a bowl and add butter, vinegar, tarragon, tomato, onion powder, garlic, salt, pepper, and stir-cook for 6 minutes to make béarnaise sauce. Cover and set aside.
3. Heat oil in another pan and fry beef until golden.
4. Cook lettuce in light salty water until wilt. Add butter and gently toss.

5. Serve beef steak over lettuce on plates and top with béarnaise sauce.

Day Fourteen

Breakfast

Western Egg Omelet

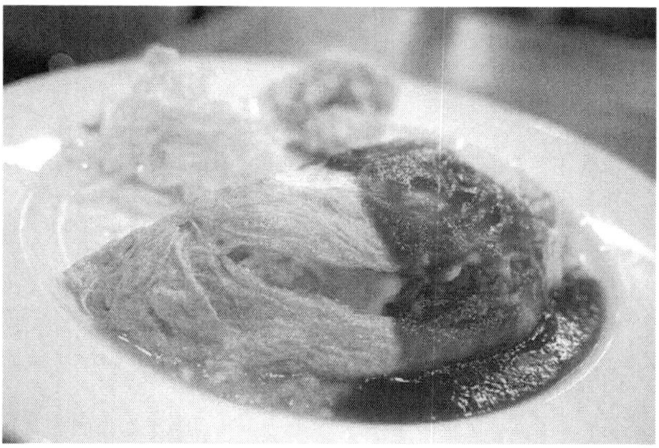

Ingredients:

1. 8 eggs.
2. 4 tbsp sour cream.

3. 1½ cup shredded cheese.
4. ½ cup unsalted butter.
5. 1 pound diced ham.
6. 1 large minced onion.
7. 1½ tsp garlic powder.
8. Salt and ground black pepper to taste.

Instruction:

1. Break eggs in a bowl. Add sour cream, half cheese, onion, garlic, salt, pepper and whisk until smooth and fluffy.
2. Melt butter in a pan and sauté diced ham.
3. Pour egg mixture into the pan with ham and fry until firm and light-golden.
4. Lower heat and pour remaining cheese and sauté until thick and crispy.

5. Serve immediately and enjoy.

Lunch

Turkey with Cream Cheese Sauce

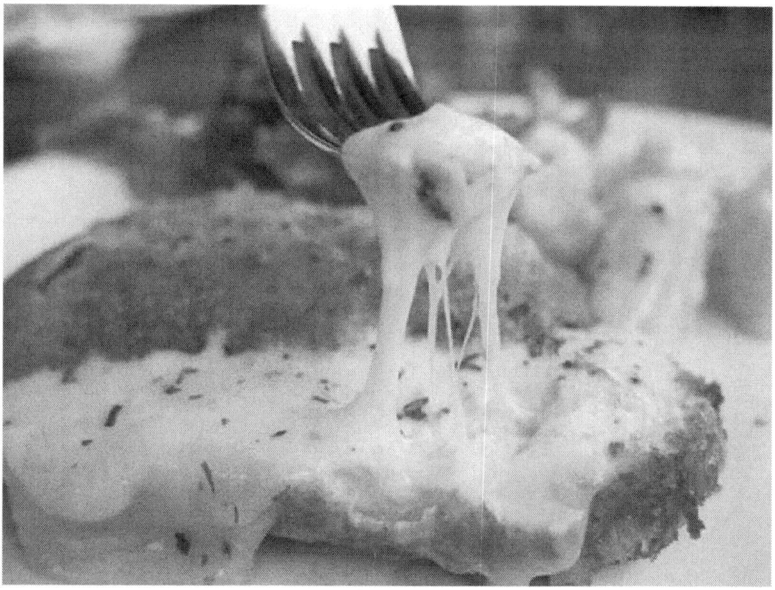

Ingredients:

1. 2 pounds fresh turkey breast.
2. 1½ cup cream cheese.

3. 2 cups whipping cream.
4. 4 unsalted tbsp butter.
5. 2 tbsp tamari soy sauce.
6. 2 tbsp dried basil.
7. 4 minced garlic cloves.
8. Salt and ground black pepper to taste.

Instruction:

1. Melt butter in pan and season turkey with salt and pepper. Sauté turkey until golden. Remove meat from pan, cover and set aside.
2. Add whipping cream and cheese into the pan and cook. Lower heat then adds basil, garlic, tamari sauce; stir and allow simmering until thick.

3. Serve turkey on plates and top with cream-cheese sauce.

Dinner: Cheeseburger with Salsa

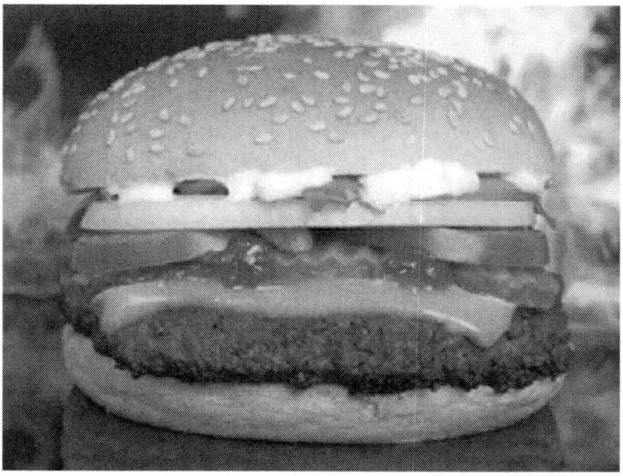

Ingredients:

1. 2pounds ground beef.
2. 2 cups shredded cheese.
3. 1 cup mayonnaise.
4. ½ cup butter.

5. 2 tbsp olive oil.
6. ½ cup dill pickle.
7. 2 avocados.
8. 4 tbsp Dijon mustard.
9. 1 pounds lettuce.
10. 4 minced tomatoes.
11. 2 large minced scallions.
12. 2½ tsp onion/garlic/paprika powder.
13. 3 tbsp minced oregano.
14. 2 tbsp minced cilantro.
15. Salt and ground black pepper to taste.

Instruction:

1. Divide avocados and fetch flesh into a bowl. Add olive oil, cilantro, scallion, tomato, salt,

pepper and stir until fluffy. Cover and set aside.

2. Pour cheese and mayonnaise in a bowl. Add onion, garlic, paprika and stir until well mixed. Add ground beef and mix until thick to form patties form frying.
3. Melt butter in a pan and fry patties until golden. Add more cheese and simmer.
4. Simmer lettuce in light salty boiling water for4 minutes and drain.
5. Serve fried cheeseburgers in plates over lettuce and top with avocado salsa, mustard and sprinkle dill pickle all over.

Part 8

CHAPTER TWELVE

Keto Smoothies and Breakfasts

A smoothie is a nutritional drink made by blending raw fruits and vegetables. Other ingredients like water, ice, yogurt, milk, and sweeteners can be added to a smoothie fruit drink. Smoothies are good for breakfast in a keto diet program. However, one should avoid much sugar in a smoothie.

Mint Smoothie

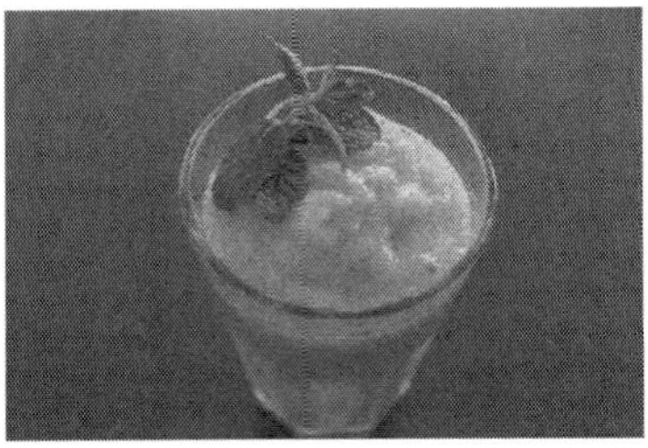

Ingredients

1. Two cups of cut baby Spinach
2. sliced spinach leaves, approximately a cup and a half of ice cubes.
3. Non-fat almondmilk
4. A half cup of packaged fresh mint leaves
5. A quarter cup of lime juice,
6. A juice of ripe mango,
7. Banana (1 if available)
8. Brown sugar 6 tablespoonsful.

Instructions

1. Blend all ingredients together and serve chilled.

Peanut Butter Cup Smoothie

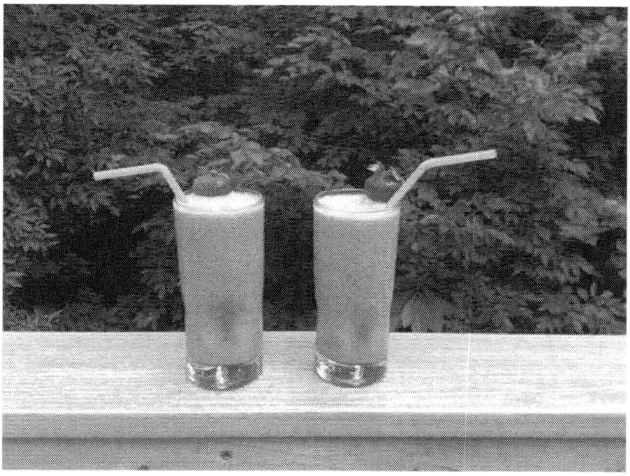

A peanut butter cup smoothie can be prepared in a different way. It depends on how you want it to look like and taste. Here is a simple way to prepare it.

Ingredients:

1. A cup of sliced ripe banana.
2. A cup of skim milk.
3. Half cup vanilla frozen yogurt.
4. 2 tbsp of peanut butter.
5. 1 vanilla yogurt.
6. Water or ice and sweeteners.

Instruction:

1. Place sliced bananas, skim milk, and vanilla yogurt in a blender and blend.
2. Add peanut butter and blend until it's thick and smooth.
3. Add some water, ice, and sweeteners as desired.

Strawberry Smoothie

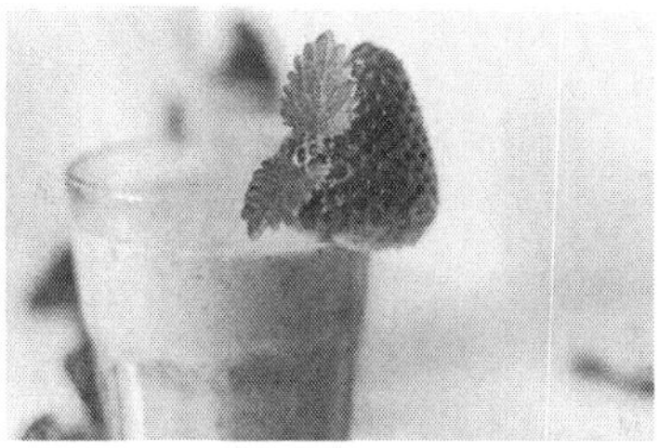

Ingredients

1. The first necessary ingredient is a quarter cup of juiced lime, brown-colored sugar 6 tablespoons
2. A half cup of mint leaves that is freshly packed, Juicy mangoes at least 1 or 2 ripe ones, One and half a cup of ice cubes, A cup of non-sweetened almondmilk, coarsely sliced 8 pieces of small strawberries.

Instructions

Blend all ingredients together and serve chilled.

Berry Green Smoothie

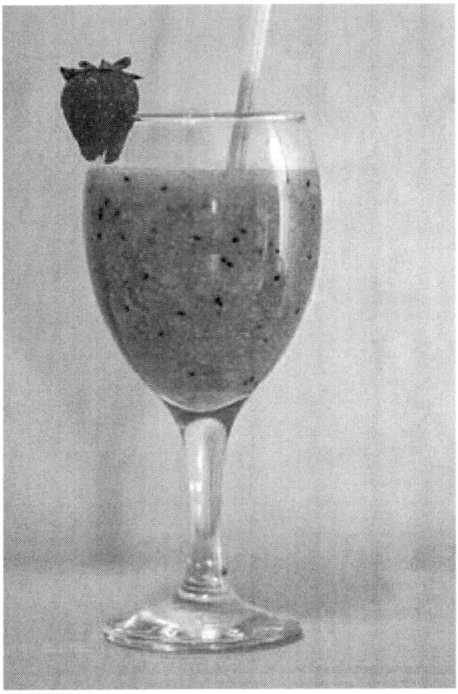

Ingredients:

1. A cup of fresh spinach leaves.
2. A half cup of frozen blueberries.
3. Half cup frozen raspberries.

4. 1 sliced banana.
5. A half cup of milk.
6. 2 tbps of oats.
7. Add sweetener to taste.

Instruction:

1. Place fresh spinach, blueberries, raspberries, banana, milk, oats in a blender and blend until smooth.
2. Add sugar and ice and blend until it's smooth.
3. Serve as desired.

Banana Smoothie

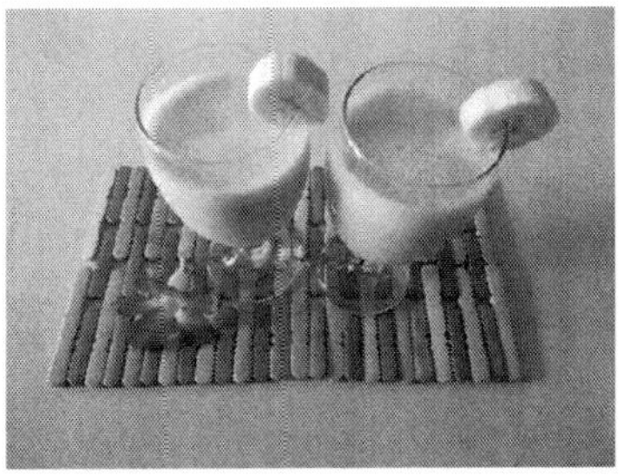

Ingredients

1. A half or 1 cup of milk
2. Banana 2 pieces
3. Cubes of ice of 5-8 (if you want).
4. A half cup of heavy organic cream,
5. 15g of honey approx 4 tbps.

Instructions

Blend all ingredients together and serve chilled.

Lemon and Cashew Smoothie

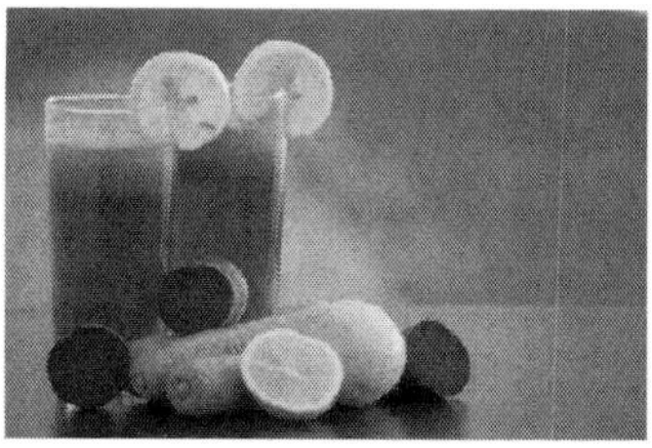

Ingredients:

1. A cup of fresh lemon juice.
2. 4 fresh raw unsalted cashews.
3. 2 sliced medium ripe banana.
4. Fresh unsweetened milk.
5. A cup of fresh vanilla yogurt.
6. Half teaspoon of lemon zest.

Instruction:

1. Place lemon juice, cashew, banana in blender and blend.

2. Add milk, vanilla yogurt, lemon zest and blend until mixture is smooth.
3. Serve as desired.

Spinach-Blueberry Smoothie

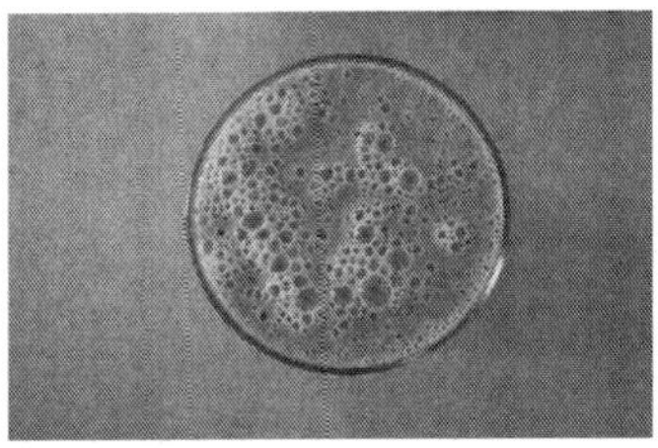

Ingredients:

1. A cup of fresh yogurt.
2. 1 sliced ripe banana.
3. A cup of fresh frozen blueberries.
4. A cup fresh spinach leaves
5. A half cup of fresh milk.

Instruction:

1. Place blueberry, spinach, banana in blender and blend.
2. Add milk and yogurt and blend until mixture is smooth.
3. Serve as desired.

Creamy Keto Cinnamon Smoothie

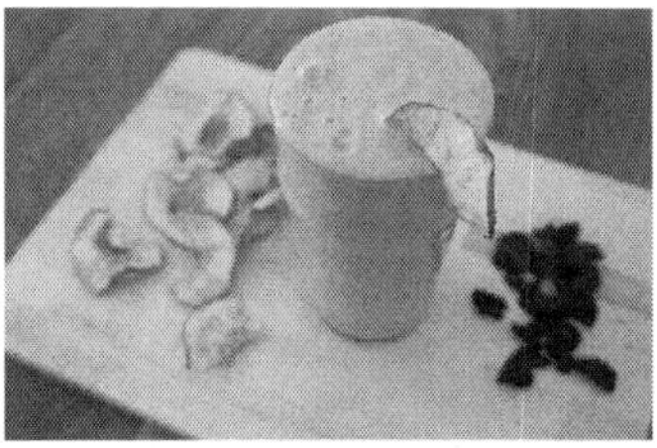

Ingredients:

1. 1 medium ripe banana.
2. 1 chopped fresh apple.
3. 2 tbsp of oats.

4. A tbsp of almond butter.
5. A cup of unsweetened milk.
6. 1 teaspoon cinnamon.
7. Water or ice.

Instruction:

1. Place banana, apple, oat, in blender and blend.
2. Add butter, milk, water, and cinnamon then blends till mixture is smooth.
3. Serve as desired.

Nut Medley Granola

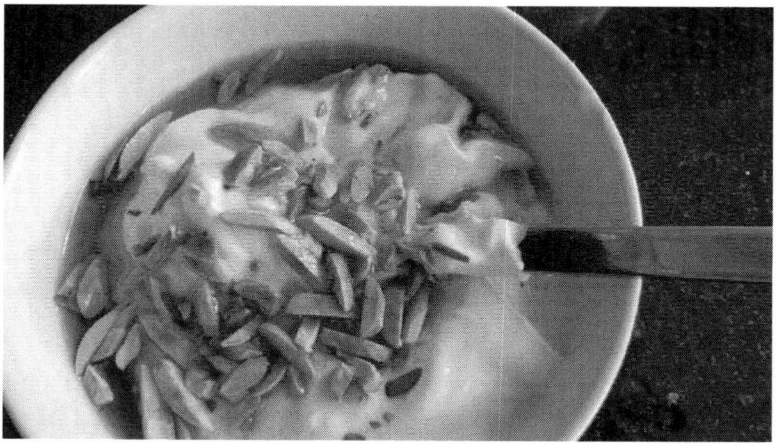

Ingredients:

1. 1 cup of chopped pecans.
2. 1 cup of chopped pistachios.
3. 1 cup of white wheat flour.
4. 3 cups of oats.
5. 2 teaspoon of cinnamon powder.
6. ½ teaspoon of salt to taste.

7. 1 cup of melted coconut oil.
8. 3 tbsp honey.

Instruction:

1. Preheat oven to 200^{oc}.
2. Mix coconut oil and honey in a bowl until smooth.
3. Add wheat flour, oat, cinnamon powder, salt, and mix.
4. Pour mixture into a large bowl. Add pecans, pistachios, and blend.
5. Pour into baking pan and bake for 1 hour stirring intermittently.
6. Remove from the oven without stirring and allow to cool.

Keto Bacon Artichoke Omelet

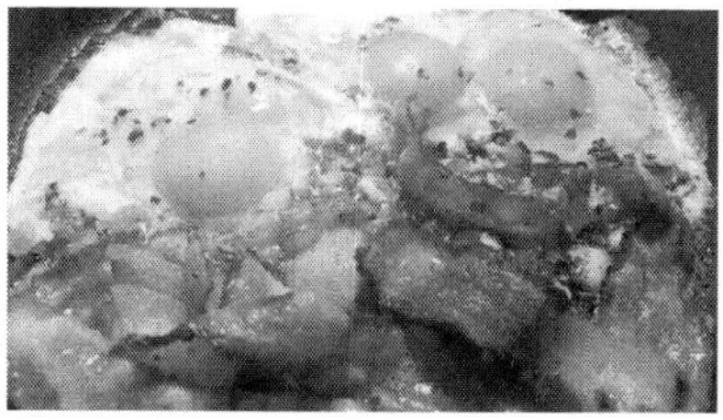

Ingredients:

1. 4 large eggs.
2. 4 large minced bacon.
3. 1 cup of cooked artichokes. Drained.
4. 1 cup of cheese
5. 1 cup of bacon broth.
6. 1 tbsp of red or black pepper.
7. 1 teaspoon of turmeric ginger.
8. Salt.

Instruction:

1. Cook bacon and then set aside to drain.
2. Put eggs in a bowl and scramble.
3. Add turmeric ginger, salt, pepper and blend.
4. Pour bacon broth in frying pan and heat. Add omelet mixture.
5. Add minced bacon, artichokes, and half cheese into omelet mixture.
6. Turn and loosen bottom of omelet using a spatula.
7. Add cheese and cook until cheese melts. Stirring mixture to blend.
8. Reduce heat and allow to cool. Serve as desired.

Keto Mushroom Frittata

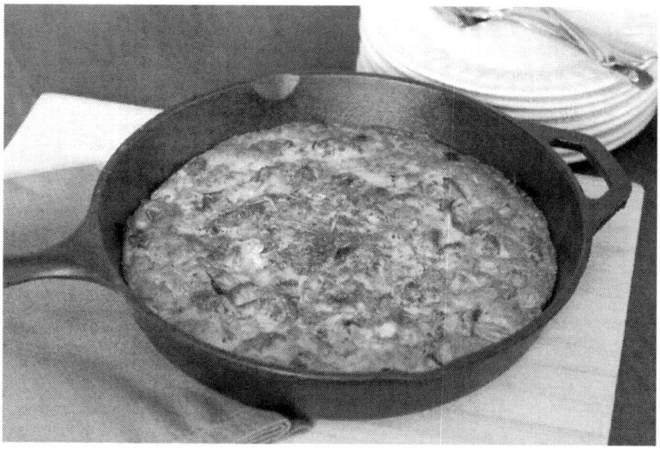

Ingredients:

1. 1 224g of the quality mushroom blend.
2. 1 cup of well-cut Parmesan pale yellow cheese.
3. 2 teaspoons of minced fresh thyme.
4. 5 large eggs.
5. Half teaspoon of salt and pepper.

Instruction:

1. Preheat frying pan at medium heat level.

2. Add mushroom and fry lightly for 10-12 minutes until it's slightly brownish.
3. Put mushroom in a bowl and let it cool. Then clean frying pan.
4. Place mushroom, cheese, thyme, eggs, salt, and pepper in a large bowl and blend with a whisk.
5. Heat frying pan again over medium heat and add whisk mushroom mixture.
6. Cover and let it cook over direct heat for 5 minutes.
7. Cut and serve as desired.

Keto Breakfast

A typical keto breakfast bake diet is that low-carb and high fat/medium protein base food. These breakfast bakes are generally known as *Keto Breakfast Casserole* like the baked or fried egg omelet, egg sausage, frittata combined with creamy cheese, milk, and avocado, etc. Vegetables like spinach, lettuce, cabbage, and mushroom can also be added to the breakfast bake. Breakfast bakes are an essential part of keto dieting. So your oven should always be available for that quick low carb breakfast bake.

Avocados and Eggs

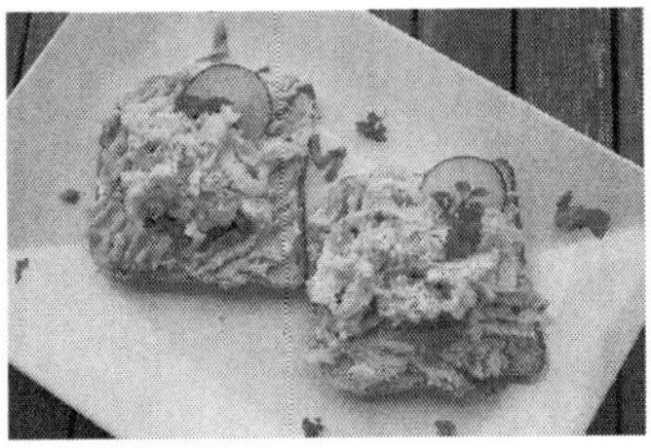

Avocados and eggs are highly nutritional low-carb food recommended for all keto dieters. Avocados produce fats and potassium that help keep the heart healthy and keep the skin fresh. Eggs, on the other hand, are rich in vitamins, minerals, and protein good for keto dieters. However, eggs could contain high cholesterol; one should avoid too much consumption.

Ingredients:

1. 2 fresh large avocados.
2. 4 eggs.
3. Sliced spring onion or normal onion.

4. 2 tbsp of mayonnaise.
5. Salt and pepper to taste.

Instruction:

1. First, boil eggs and apply a small pinch of salt to avoid cracking.
2. Remove egg shells and cut eggs into pieces and place in a bowl.
3. Divide avocados and remove the seeds then fetch half of the cream flesh and place inside the bowl containing cut egg pieces.
4. Add mayonnaise, onion, pepper, and salt into the bowl and mix with egg and avocado cream until well mixed.

5. Fetch from the bowl and serve with divided avocado.

Part 9

CHAPTER THIRTEEN

Apps and Snacks

Apps are appetizer meals served before main meal course to stimulate and boost one's appetite. Snacks, on the other hand, are easy to prepare meals eaten in-between main meals. Keto dieters should always consume specially prepared low-carb apps and snacks.

Ketogenic Diet Bacon Pepper Fat Bombs:

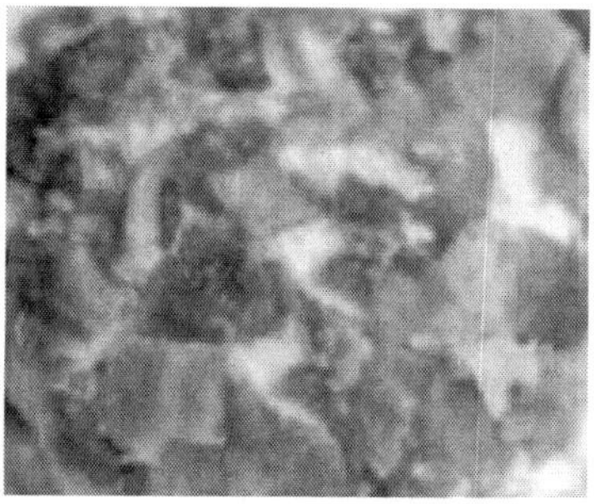

Ingredients:

1. 6 large slices of fresh bacon.
2. 4 large eggs.
3. 2 tbsp of mayonnaise.
4. Fresh pepper powder.
5. Half teaspoon of salt to taste.

Instruction:

1. Preheat oven to 200^{oc} and then place bacon on baking paper and cook for 12-15 minutes till it turns light brown then remove to cool.

2. Boil eggs with some salt to prevent cracking for 15 minutes then put in a bowl to cool.
3. Slice egg into small pieces then pours into bacon grease. Add mayonnaise, pepper, and salt and mix.
4. Put in the fridge until it's solid to form fat bombs.
5. Break bacon into tiny bits and start forming balls using egg mixture from fridge.
6. Serve immediately as desired.

Smoked Salmon Keto Fat Bombs

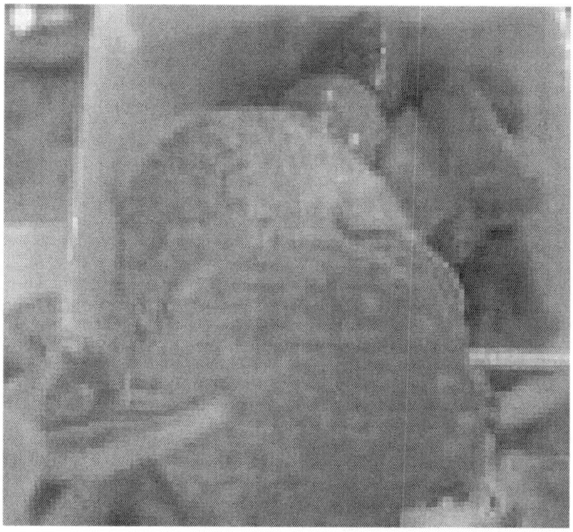

Ingredients:

1. 1 pack of smoked salmon fish.
2. 1 cup of fresh cream cheese.
3. A half cup of butter.
4. 1 tbsp of fresh lemon juice.
5. 1-2 tbsp freshly minced dill.
6. 1 teaspoon of salt and pepper.

Instruction:

1. Place salmon fish in a blender or mixer.
2. Add cream cheese and butter and start blending.
3. Add fresh lemon juice and dill. Keep blending until smooth.
4. Create small fat bombs fetching 2 or 3 tablespoons from the mixture and line in a tray.
5. Put in the fridge for 1-2 hours until bombs are firm.
6. Serve immediately as desired.

Keto Walnut Herb-Crusted Goat Cheese

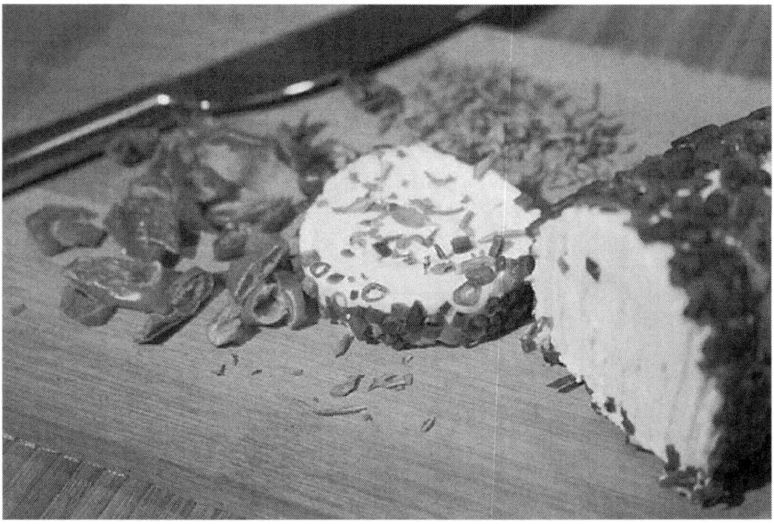

Ingredients:

1. 6 pieces of fresh walnut.
2. 1 medium pack of fresh goat cheese.
3. 2 fresh bunches of shredded beetroot.
4. 4 tbsp of well minced parsley leaves.
5. 2 tbsp of sliced mint leaves and thyme.
6. 2 small crushed garlic clove.

7. 2 tbsp of vinegar.
8. 4 tbsp of pure olive oil.
9. 4-6 slice of bread.

Instruction:

1. Preheat oven to 200^{oc} then wrap beetroots and thyme. Then bake for 40 minutes, and then allow to cool.
2. Put walnut pieces on a baking tray and bake for 8 minutes till it turns golden brown.
3. Crush walnut and then add parsley and mint leaves and blend. Add cheese and blend on.
4. Cut bread into cube size and then toss with crushed garlic. Add 1 tbsp of olive oil and then

bake for 10 minutes until it turns golden brown.

5. Mix remaining olive oil with vinegar and whisk in a bowl.
6. Add walnut and other mixtures and then serve from mixtures as desired.

Keto Crispy Parmesan Crackers

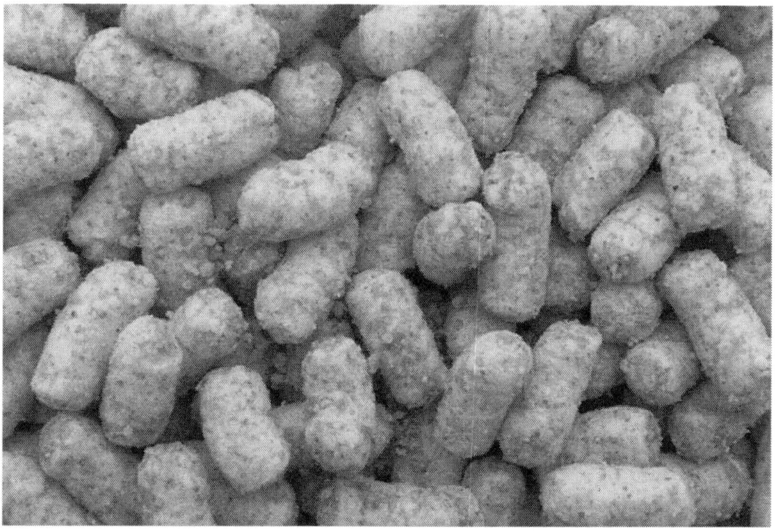

Ingredients:

1. 1 cup of grated Parmesan cheese.
2. 4 cups of wheat flour.
3. 1 cup of milk.
4. 4 tbsp of butter.
5. 2 teaspoon of fresh black pepper powder.
6. Half teaspoon of salt.

Instruction:

1. Pour wheat flour in a bowl and mix with butter and parmesan cream cheese.
2. Add salt and pepper and blend the mixture until it turns into dough.
3. Join dough balls together and then flatten dough with a clean bottle.
4. Divide flat dough into small squares for baking.
5. Bake for 15-20 minutes until dough turns golden brown.

Keto Bacon Cheese Deviled Eggs

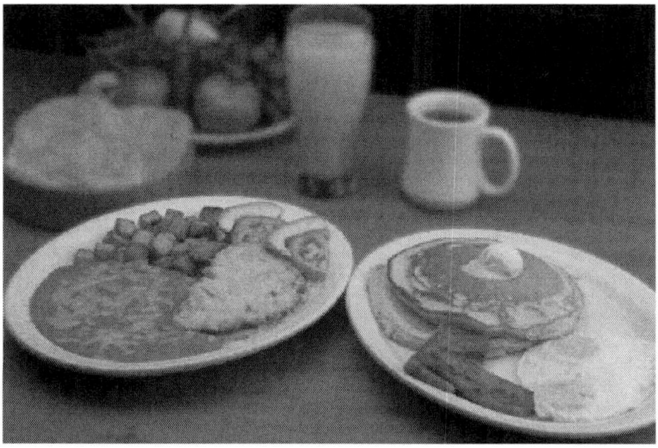

Ingredients:

1. 10 large cooked eggs, peeled.
2. A half cup of fresh cheese.
3. 5 large slice of cooked bacon. Shred.
4. A half cup of mayonnaise.
5. 1 teaspoon black pepper.
6. 2 tbsp minced cheddar.
7. Fresh parsley leaves to garnish.
8. Half teaspoon of salt.

Instruction:

1. Divide cooked eggs into two equal halves.
2. Fetch out yolks using a spoon into a bowl and keep whites.
3. Place shred bacon in a bowl and blend with cheese.
4. Crush yolks with a spoon and add mayonnaise, cheddar, salt, and pepper. Blend mixture.
5. Fill each half egg white with yolk mixture and garnish with parsley.
6. Cover and put in fridge until ready to serve.

Queso Dip

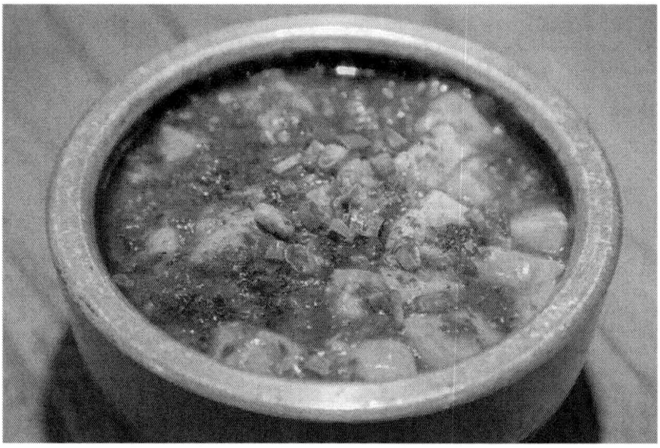

Ingredients:

1. 2 cans of undrained tomatoes.
2. Fresh green chilies.
3. 1 teaspoon of red and black pepper.
4. Half teaspoon of cumin.
5. Half teaspoon of jalapeno
6. Velveeta cubed cheese.
7. Salt.

Instruction:

1. Place undrained tomatoes and Velveeta cheese in a saucepan and blend.
2. Add chilies, pepper, cumin and jalapeno and blend mixture.
3. Cook over medium heat and stir frequently until mixture is blended.
4. Serve warm as a dip with tortilla chips, crackers or cut-up fresh vegetables.

Ketogenic Diet Cauliflower-Cheddar Soup

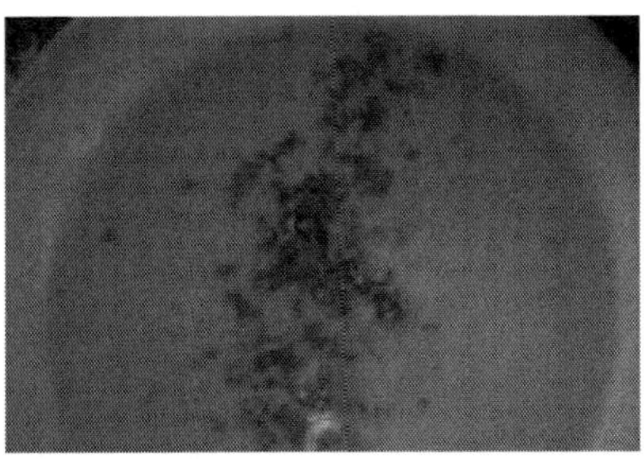

Ingredients:

1. 4 tablespoons of butter. Unsalted.

2. 1 large diced onion.
3. 1 large cauliflower head. Sliced.
4. 4 cups of hot chicken broth.
5. 5 ounce of grated white cheddar.
6. 1 teaspoon of cayenne pepper.
7. $^1/_2$ teaspoon of salt to taste.

Instruction:

1. Put butter in a pot and melt with onion over medium heat. Stir occasionally.
2. Add cauliflower and cook until is begin to turn brown then add chicken broth with small water and boil until cauliflower becomes soft.
3. Simmer the mixture for a while then pour into a large bowl.

4. Pour mixture into a blender and blend until smooth.
5. Pour back mixture into the pot and add more chicken broth, pepper, cayenne, and salt then cook over low heat.
6. Increase heat and add cheddar cheese and stir until it melts.
7. Serve immediately as desired.

Bacon, Lettuce and Tomato Salad (BLT)

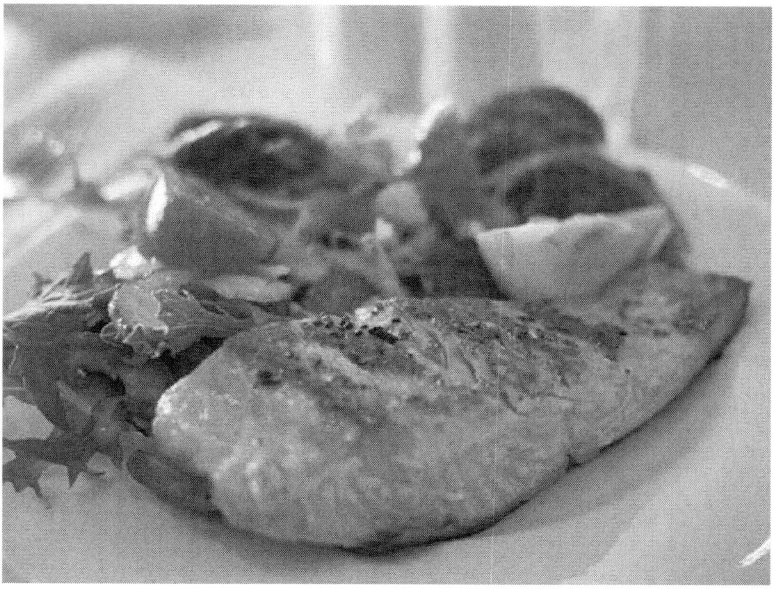

Ingredients:

9. 5 large shredded bacon.
10. 2 heads of fresh lettuce. Sliced.
11. 4 large tomatoes. Sliced.
12. 1 cup of milk.
13. ½ cup of mayonnaise.
14. 1 teaspoon of garlic powder.

15.1 teaspoon of black pepper powder.

16. Salt to taste.

Instruction:

6. Cook shredded bacon over medium heat until it turns brownish.
7. Place milk, mayonnaise, garlic and pepper in a blender and blend until smooth.
8. Place tomatoes, lettuce, and bacon in a bowl.
9. Pour blended content into the bowl containing tomatoes, lettuce, and bacon and blend together.
10. Serve immediately as desired.

Chicken-Avocado Lettuce Wrap

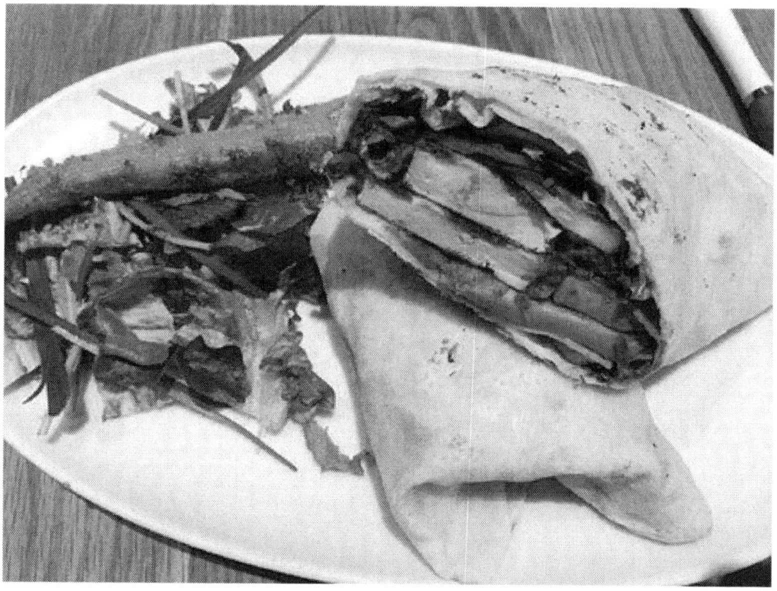

Ingredients:

1. 4 large shredded chicken meat.
2. 1 head of fresh lettuce. Remove leaves apart.
3. 2 large avocados.
4. 3 tbsp olive oil.
5. 3 tbsp lime juice.

6. 1 tbsp garlic powder.
7. 2 tbsp chopped fresh cilantro leaves.
8. 2 teaspoon of pepper powder.
9. Salt.

Instruction:

1. Preheat oven to 160^{oc}.
2. Rub olive oil on the chicken meat and sprinkle lime juice seasoning all over.
3. Place chicken meat in a shallow baking dish and bake meat in the preheated oven. Then remove from oven and let it cool.
4. Place chicken in a large bowl and then add avocado flesh, lime juice, cilantro, garlic powder, salt, pepper and mix well.

5. Serve on top of lettuce leaves to make wraps.

Crab Salad Stuffed Avocado

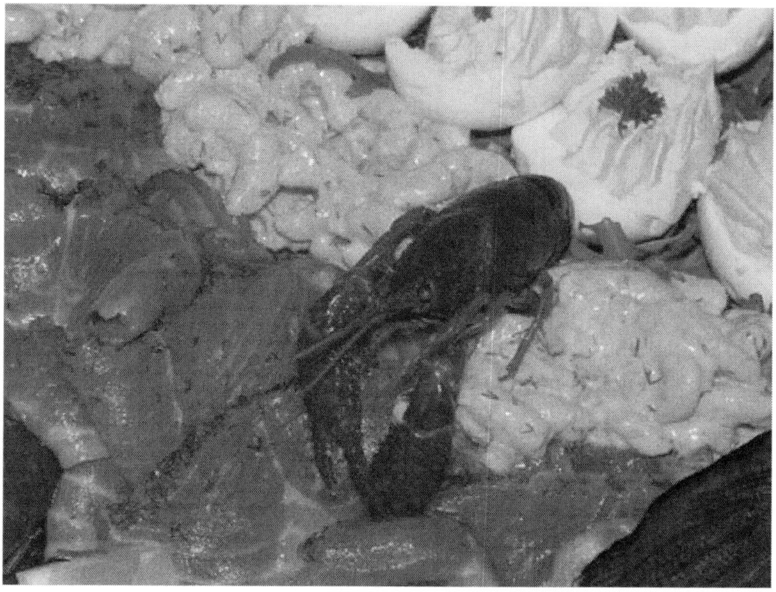

Ingredients:

1. 2 large ripe avocados.
2. 6 oz shredded crab meat.
3. 2 fresh large minced lettuce leaves.

4. 3 fresh minced tomatoes.
5. 2 tbsp chopped cilantro leaves.
6. 2 tbsp olive oil.
7. 4 tbsp lime juice.
8. 2 tbsp minced onion.
9. 1 tbsp pepper powder.
10. 1/2 teaspoon of salt.

Instruction:

1. Place olive oil, onion, lime juice, cilantro, lettuce and tomato in a bowl and blend.
2. Add cooked crab meat, pepper, salt, and toss.
3. Divide avocado into equal halves and remove seed.

4. Use a spoon to fetch half of the flesh. Put into a bowl with crab salad mixture and toss.
5. Fill each avocado have with crab salad and serve.

Part 10

CHAPTER FOURTEEN

VEGETABLES AND SIDES

Vegetables are plants with fresh edible leafy parts that are eaten in food or specially prepared as salads. Some vegetables are consumed raw while some are cooked before consuming. Vegetables are good appetizers and body builders. Vegetables are also meals for Vegetarians; however, Keto dieters are advised to consume a lot of vegetables.

Portobello Mushroom Pizza

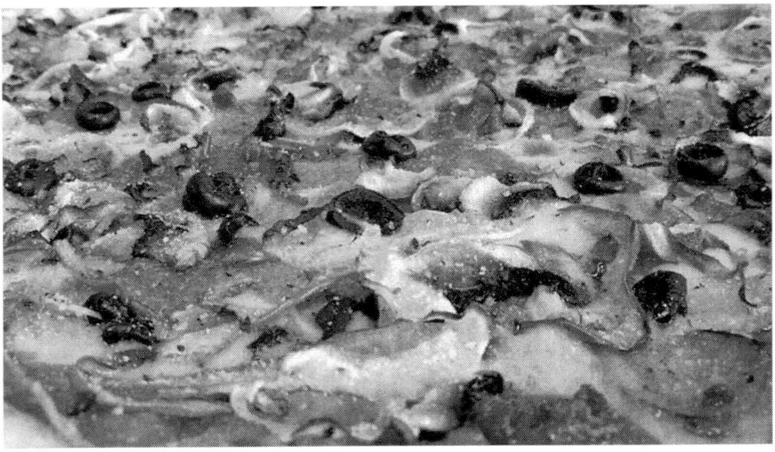

Ingredients:

1. 6 large Portobello mushroom caps. Remove stems.
2. 4 large minced tomato.
3. 3 cups shredded Italian white cheese.
4. 4 tbsp virgin olive oil.
5. ½ cup finely minced parsley.
6. ½ cup finely minced basil.
7. Salt and pepper to taste.

Instruction:

1. Preheat oven to 180^{oc}.
2. Cook mushroom until nearly done. Set aside and allow to drain.
3. Coat mushroom caps with olive oil and season with salt and pepper.
4. Place mushroom in a baking dish and add cheese, tomato, parsley, basil and toast mixture gently.
5. Put into oven and bake for 25-30 minutes until mushroom is done and cheese melts.
6. Remove and serve immediately.

Garlicky Green Beans

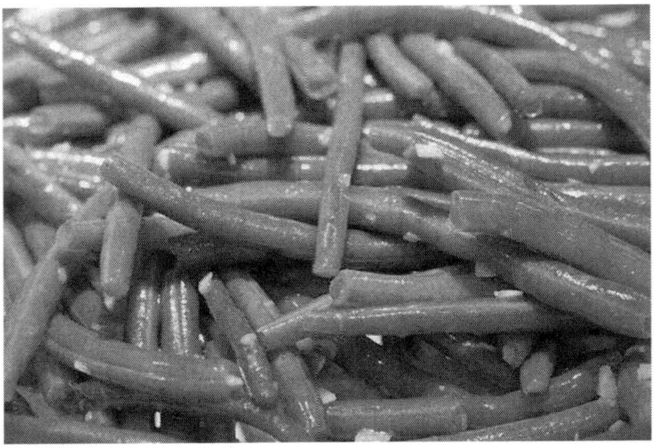

Ingredients:

1. 4 pounds fresh finely trimmed green beans.
2. 8 finely minced garlic cloves.
3. ½ cup extra virgin olive oil.
4. 4 tbsp finely minced parsley.
5. 2 tbsp dried tarragon leaves.
6. 1 tbsp pepper powder.
7. 1 tsp salt to taste.

Instruction:

1. Cook green beans in boiling water for 6 minutes until soft. Set aside to drain and cool.
2. Heat oil in a pan over medium heat; add garlic and stir-cook for 1 minute.
3. Add green beans, parsley, tarragon, pepper, salt, and stir.
4. Stir-cook for 6 minutes. Set aside and allow to cool.
5. Serve immediately as desired.

Sauced Asparagus with Walnuts

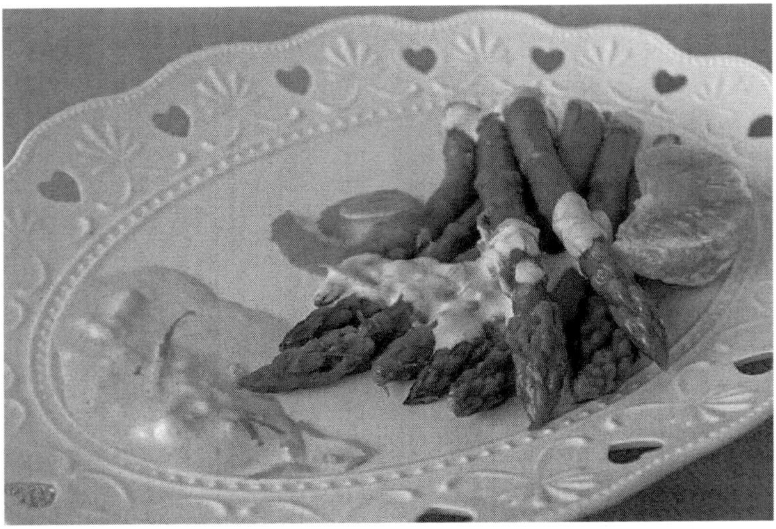

Ingredients:

1. 2 pounds fresh asparagus. Cut out hard ends.
2. 1 cup finely chopped walnut.
3. 1 tbsp walnut oil.
4. 1 cup soybeans cream.
5. ½ cup soy sauce.
6. Salt and pepper to taste.

Instruction:

1. Cook asparagus in a light salty boiling water until soft.
2. Heat oil in a pan. Add walnuts and stir-fry for 4 minutes.
3. Reduce heat and add soybeans cream/sauce. Stir and allow to cook.
4. Add salt and pepper.
5. Serve cooked asparagus on plates and top with walnut sauce.

Brussels Sprout Casserole

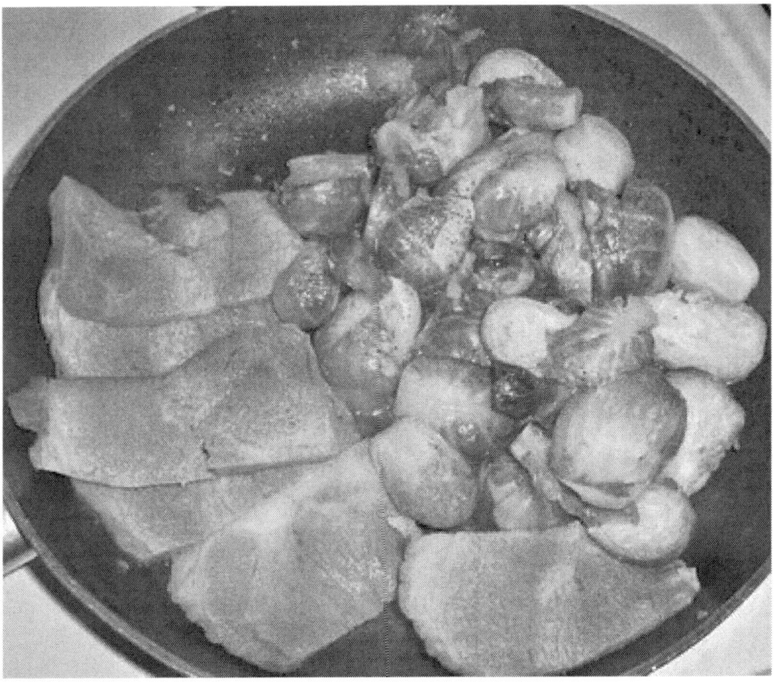

Ingredients:

1. 4 pounds Brussels sprouts. Divide into equal halves.
2. ½ cup butter.
3. 3 finely minced shallot bulb.
4. 1 cup grated white cheese.

5. 1 cup crumbled cooked bacon.
6. 1 cup fresh cream.
7. 1 tsp red pepper.
8. Salt.

Instruction:

1. Preheat oven to 190^{oc}.
2. Melt butter in a large pan.
3. Add Brussels sprout and shallot. Add salt and red pepper and allow to cook for 12 minutes until soft. Stir occasionally.
4. Reduce heat and pour cream. Add cheese and bacon and toast.
5. Bake for 16 minutes until cheese melts. Remove and set aside to cool.
6. Serve immediately as desired.

Creamed Spinach

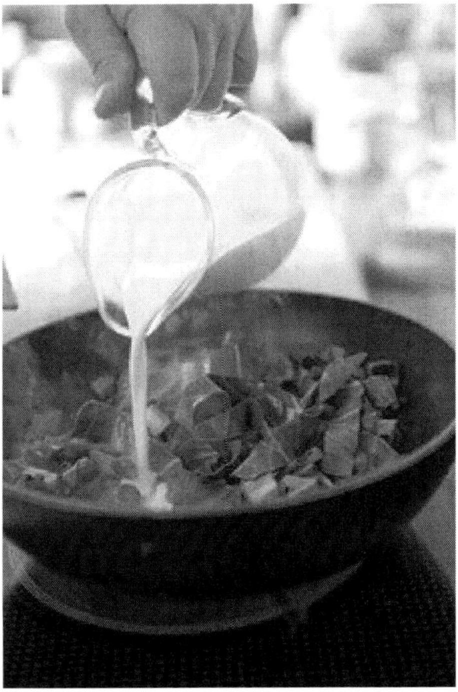

Ingredients:

1. 4 pounds finely minced spinach.
2. ½ butter.
3. 1 large finely minced onion.
4. 6 finely minced garlic cloves.

5. 1 cup shredded cream cheese.
6. 1 cup fresh milk.
7. Salt and pepper powder to taste.

Instruction:

1. Cook spinach in lightly salted boiling water until soft. Set aside, pour cold water to cool, then drain properly.
2. Heat butter in a large pan until it melts.
3. Over medium heat, add garlic, onion, pepper, salt, and stir-cook for 6 minutes.
4. Add milk and cheese and stir-cook until cheese melts.
5. Pour spinach into cheese mixture, stir and add little pepper and salt. Let it simmer for 10 minutes.

6. Serve immediately as desired.

Cheesy Mashed Cauliflower

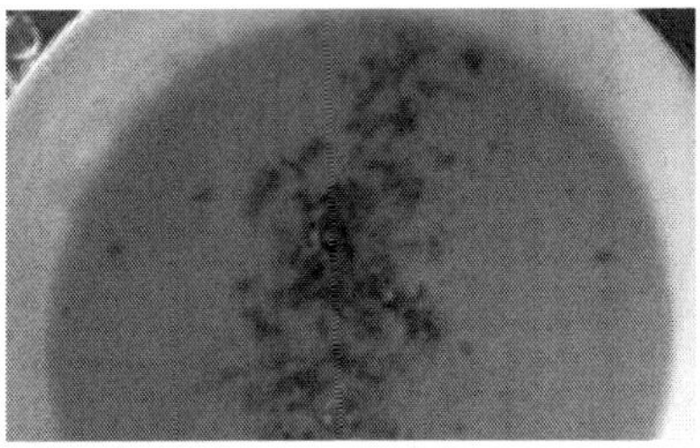

Ingredients:

1. 2 pounds cauliflower head. Trimmed.
2. 1 cup cheddar cheese. Grated.
3. ½ cup cream cheese.
4. ½ butter.
5. 4 finely minced garlic cloves.
6. Salt and ground pepper to taste.

Instruction:

1. Preheat oven to 200^{oc}.
2. Trim cauliflower and cut into medium size florets.
3. Cook cauliflower over medium heat in lightly salted boiling water for 10 minutes until soft. Then set aside to drain.
4. Melt butter in hot pan. Add cheddar cheese and cook until it melts.
5. Reduce heat and add cream cheese, garlic, pepper, and salt. Stir and allow to cook until smooth.
6. Pour cauliflower into cheese mixture and toast.

7. Place mixture into a baking casserole and bake for 15 minutes.
8. Serve immediately as desired.

Sautéed Crispy Zucchini

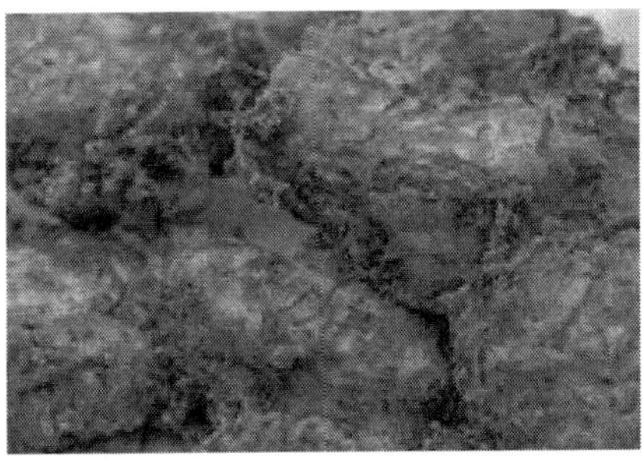

Ingredients:

1. 2 pounds finely trimmed zucchini.
2. 1 cup finely grated parmesan cheese.
3. 2 tbsp extra virgin olive oil.
4. 2 finely minced garlic cloves.
5. 1 tbsp minced red pepper.

6. Salt and black pepper to taste.

Instruction:

1. Heat oil in large pan. Add garlic and red pepper and stir-cook for 40 seconds.
2. Add zucchini, toast in oil and allow to cook until golden brown.
3. Add parmesan cheese, pepper, salt and allow to cook until cheese melts.
4. Serve immediately as desired.

Mushroom with Camembert

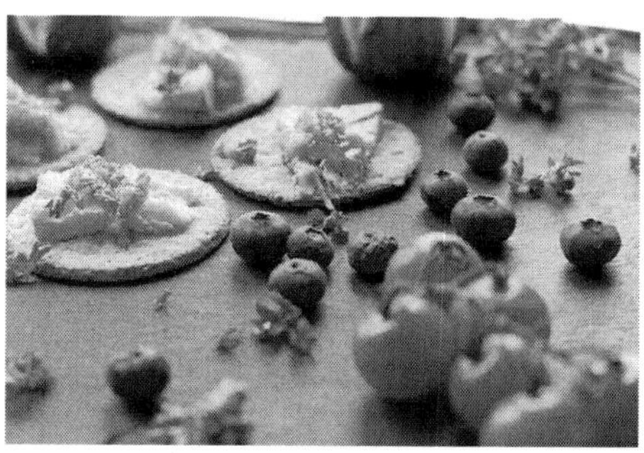

Ingredients:

1. 5 large Portobello mushroom. Remove stems.
2. 2 cup shredded French camembert.
3. 2 medium size finely minced shallot.
4. 4 finely minced garlic cloves.
5. ½ cup olive oil.
6. 4 sprigs of thyme. Minced.
7. Salt and ground pepper to taste.

Instruction:

1. Preheat oven to 200^{oc}.
2. Wash mushroom and cook in salty boiling water until soft. Drain well and set aside to cool.

3. Heat oil in a large pan. Add mushroom and cook for 4 minutes until brownish. Set mushroom aside.
4. Return pan with oil to heat. Add shallot, garlic, thyme and sauté for 4 minutes then add camembert, pepper, and salt. Toast mixture and allow to cook until camembert melts.
5. Pour mixture into baking pan and bake in preheated oven for 15-20 minutes until golden brown.
6. Serve immediately as desired.

Pesto Zucchini Noodles

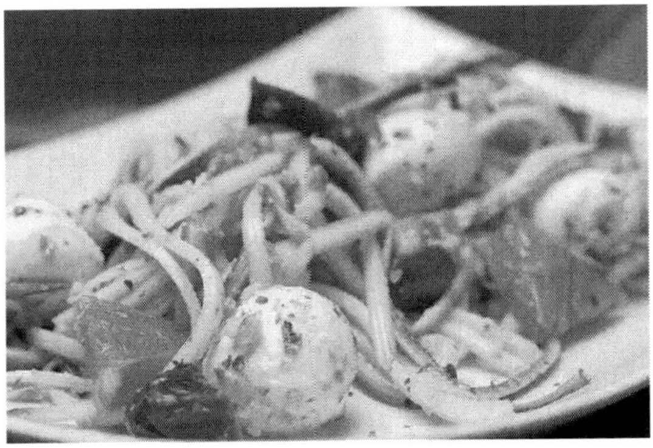

Ingredients:

1. 2 pounds zucchini. Trim ends.
2. 1 cup finely grated parmesan cheese.
3. ½ cup fresh lemon juice.
4. ½ cup virgin olive oil.
5. 4 finely minced garlic cloves.
6. 4 tbsp finely minced basil leaves.
7. 4 finely minced tomato.
8. Salt and ground pepper to taste.

Instruction:

1. Slice trimmed zucchini into noodles using a peeler.
2. Heat oil in a large pan. Add garlic and basil and stir-cook for 2 minutes.
3. Add zucchini noodles. Season with salt and pepper; toast and cook until half done.
4. Add parmesan cheese and lemon juice and cook until cheese melt. Reduce heat.
5. Add tomato, and little more pepper and salt then simmer for 6-8 minutes.
6. Serve immediately as desired.

Golden Rosti

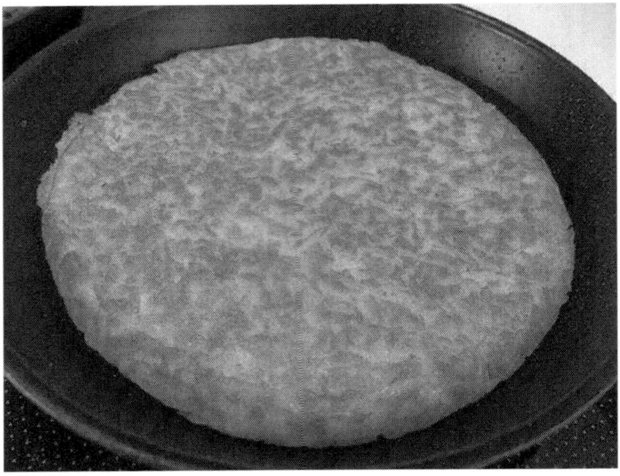

Ingredients:

1. 2 pound fresh grated potatoes. Peeled.
2. 1 pounds shredded bacon.
3. 1 large finely minced onion
4. 2 finely minced garlic cloves.
5. 4 tbsp butter.
6. Salt and ground pepper to taste.

Instruction:

1. Cook potatoes in boiling water until nearly done. Drain and set aside.
2. Melt butter in a large pan. Add garlic and onion and stir-fry for 1 minute.
3. Add potatoes and coat with butter then add salt and pepper and toast to combine.
4. Add bacon, stir and cook for 20-25 minutes until crisp and golden brown.
5. Serve immediately as desired.

CHAPTER FIFTEEN

KETO FISH AND POULTRY

Fish and poultry products are essential meals for keto dieters. These products are rich in fats and oil to help trigger and quicken your transition to that ketotic state as quick as possible. Fish and poultry meals come in a wide variety depending on how you want it. Be sure to look out for high fat fish and poultry products for your keto diets. Here and some recipes.

Seared Shrimp and Sausage

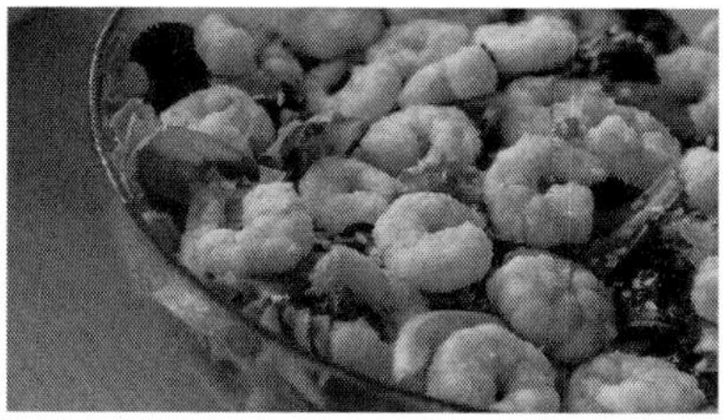

Ingredients:

1. 1 package of sliced smoked sausage.
2. 2 pounds of deveined shrimp.
3. 4 big peeled potatoes. Sliced.
4. 1/2 cup of melt unsalted butter.
5. 4 cloves of minced garlic.
6. 2 tbsp of fresh minced parsley.
7. 1 teaspoon of salt and 1 tbsp of pepper.

Instruction:

1. Preheat oven to 190^{oc}.

2. Cook potato in salted water for 10-15 minutes. Set aside and drain.
3. Put butter, garlic, pepper, and salt in a bowl and blend.
4. Add shrimp, sausage, and potato into butter mixture and toss for baking.
5. Bake in the oven for 15-20 minutes then serve with parsley leaves to garnish.

Herb Butter Scallop

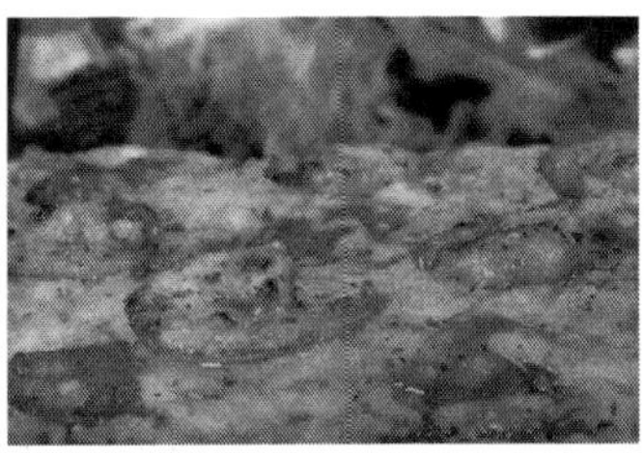

Ingredients:

1. 2 pounds of fresh sea scallop.

2. 4 sprigs minced parsley, oregano or thyme herb.
3. 4 tbsp of unsalted brown butter.
4. 3 tbsp of lemon juice.
5. 2 tbsp of olive oil.
6. Salt and black pepper powder.

Instruction:

1. Heat oil over medium heat in a pan.
2. Wash scallop and add pepper and salt.
3. Cook scallops for 8-10 minutes until it turns golden-brown.
4. Add butter and herbs to skillet and stir at intervals until scallop is well cooked and butter melts.

5. Add lemon juice and toss. Then serve.

Halibut sauced with Citrus Butter

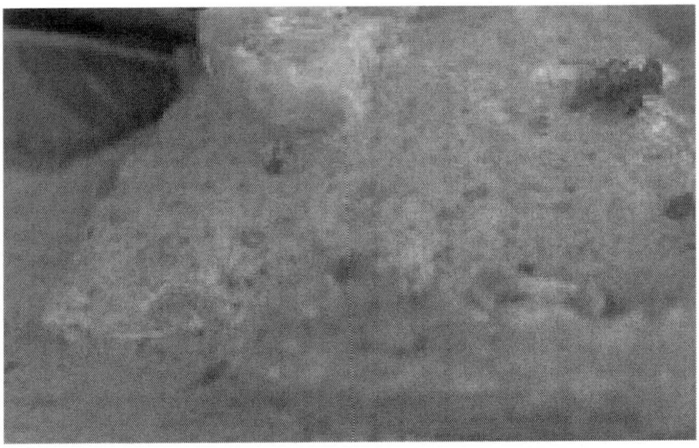

Ingredients:

1. 2 pound fresh halibut sea fish.
2. 1 cup of citrus juice.
3. 1 cup of white flour.
4. 1 tbsp of sliced shallot or 1 tbsp of onion powder.

5. 1 tbsp of slice garlic.
6. 1 tbsp of black pepper.
7. 1 tbsp of sliced parsley, thyme or oregano.
8. 1 cup of cooking wine.
9. 1/2 of butter and cream.
10. 3 tbsp olive oil.
11. 1 tsp salt to taste.

Instruction:

1. Put oil in a pan and warm over medium heat.
2. Fry halibut in oil for 6-8 minutes.
3. Pour cooking wine into a large pan and warm over medium heat.

4. Increase heat and add citrus juice, garlic, pepper, shallot, onion powder, parsley, thyme, oregano, and blend.
5. Reduce heat and add flour, cream, and butter. Blend to form citrus butter sauce.
6. Server fried halibut in plates and put citrus butter sauce as desired. Add fresh parsley on top to garnish.

Fish Curry

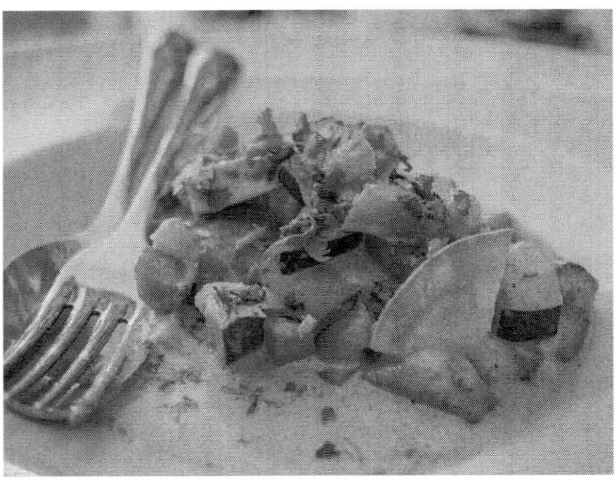

Ingredients:

1. 2 pounds fresh fish.
2. 2 tbsp vegetable oil.
3. 1 medium size sachet tomato paste.
4. 1 large minced onion.
5. 4 minced garlic clove.
6. 1 tbsp minced curry leaves.
7. 1 tbsp curry paste or powder.
8. 1 tbsp pepper and 1 tsp salt to taste.

Instruction:

1. Cook fish with some salt and spice over medium heat until half done.
2. Heat oil in a deep frying pan over medium heat.

3. Add minced onion and garlic and fry for 4 minutes.
4. Add curry paste and tomato paste and stir-fry for a while.
5. Add fish with broth to curry paste mixture. Then add curry leaves, pepper, salt and cook till fish is fully done.
6. Serve immediately as desired.

Roasted Salmon with Avocado Salsa

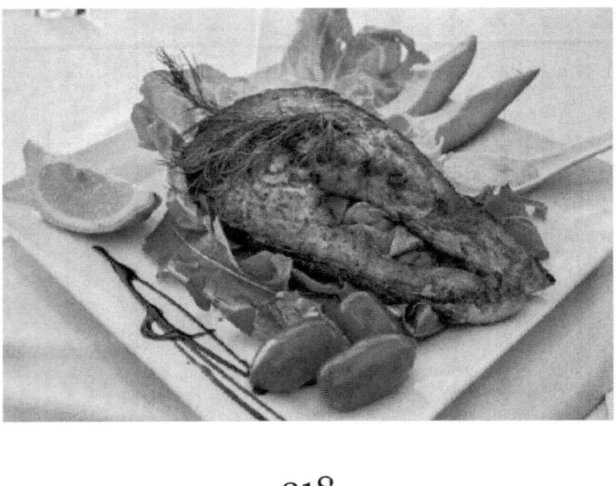

Ingredients:

1. 3 pounds of boneless salmon.
2. 2 medium size ripe avocados.
3. 1 small head of finely minced lettuce.
4. 2 tsp paprika
5. 2 tsp garlic and onion powder.
6. 1 large finely minced onion.
7. 2 tbsp avocado oil.
8. 4 tbsp lime juice.
9. 2 tbsp minced cilantro leaves.
10. Salt and pepper to taste.

Instruction:

1. Preheat oven to 190^{oc}.
2. Apply small avocado oil to grease baking pan.
3. Divide avocados, remove flesh and put in a bowl. Add avocado oil, lime juice, cilantro, minced onion, and lettuce. Toss to make avocado salsa.
4. Cover mixture and refrigerate for 1 hour or more.
5. Place salmon on a baking pan and rub garlic and onion powder, paprika all over.
6. Put baking pan in the oven and bake for 18-20 minutes.

Sole Asiago

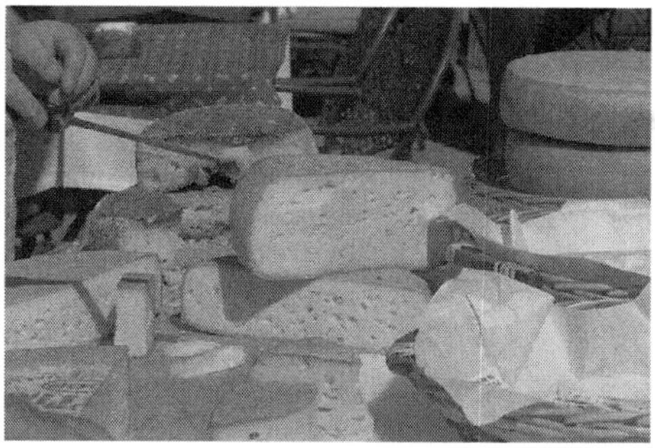

Ingredients:

1. 1 cup of shredded asiago cheese.
2. $^1/_2$ cup of goat cheese.
3. 2 pounds freshly shredded bacon.
4. 4 finely sliced garlic clove.
5. 1 cup of white flour.
6. 3 eggs
7. $^1/_2$ cup of vegetable oil.
8. 1 tsp salt and 2 tsp pepper powder.

Instruction:

1. Preheat oven to 200°C.
2. Cook bacon over medium heat until almost done. Set aside to cool.
3. In a deep bowl, mix asiago cheese, goat cheese, pepper, salt and then refrigerate for 1 hour or more.
4. Mix flour and egg with some cheese and oil.
5. Mix flour mixture with asiago cheese mixture and shredded bacon.
6. Flatten with a bottle and cut into the desired shape.
7. Put into baking pan and bake for 30-40 minutes.

Baked Coconut Keto Haddock

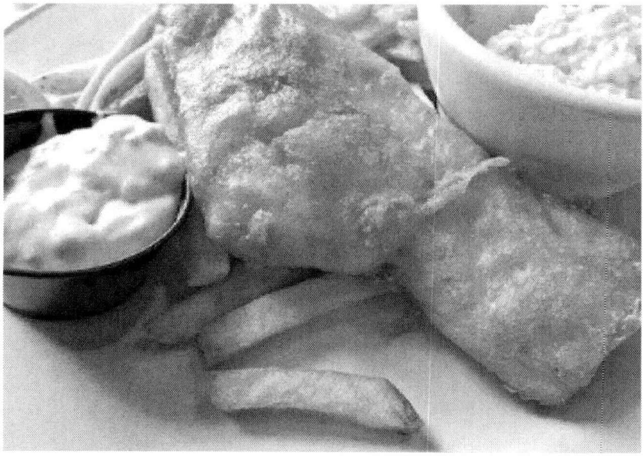

Ingredients:

1. 2 pounds fillet of haddock.
2. 1 cup of shredded fresh coconut.
3. 4 beaten eggs.
4. 1 cup of wheat breadcrumbs.
5. $^1/_2$ teaspoon nutmeg.
6. ½ cup of crushed macadamia nut.
7. Salt and pepper to taste.

Instruction:

1. Preheat oven to 180^{oc}.
2. Place breadcrumb in a large bowl; add coconut, nutmeg, macadamia nut, salt, and pepper. Blend.
3. Pour beaten eggs into a different bowl and coat haddock fillets with egg.
4. Also, coat haddock fillets with breadcrumb mixture.
5. Place baking sheet on baking pan and place coated haddock fillets.
6. Put into oven and bake for 20-30minutes.

Cheesy Garlic Salmon

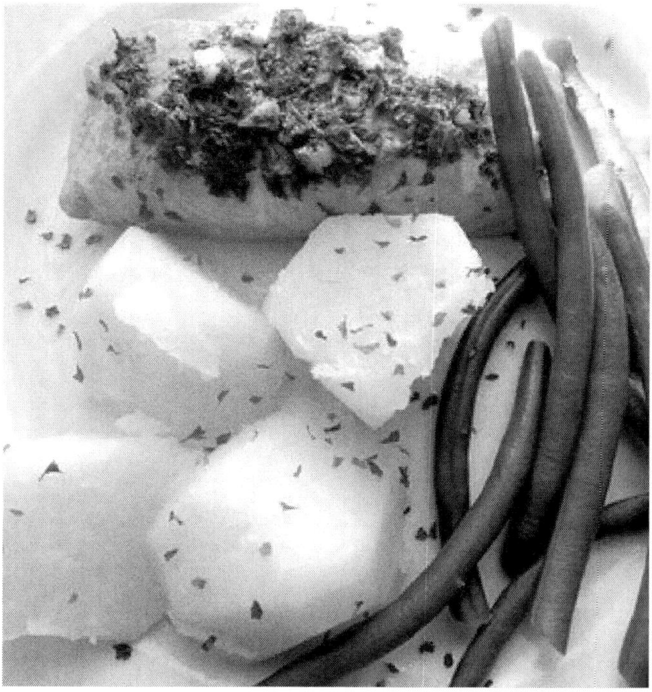

Ingredients:

1. 4 pounds fresh salmon fillets.
2. 1 cup of shredded parmesan cheese.
3. ½ cup of melted butter.
4. 6 finely minced garlic cloves.
5. ½ cup finely minced parsley leaves.
6. 1 cup of wheat breadcrumbs.
7. Salt and pepper to taste.

Instruction:

1. Preheat oven to 190^{oc}.
2. Place breadcrumb in a large bowl. Add cheese, melted butter, parsley, garlic, pepper, salt and mix until well mixed with breadcrumb.
3. Place baking sheet on a baking tray and place salmon fillets on.
4. Coat salmon fillets with breadcrumb-cheese mixture.
5. Put into oven and bake for 10-15 minutes until it turns golden brown.
6. Serve as desired with salad or vegetables.

Lemon Butter Chicken

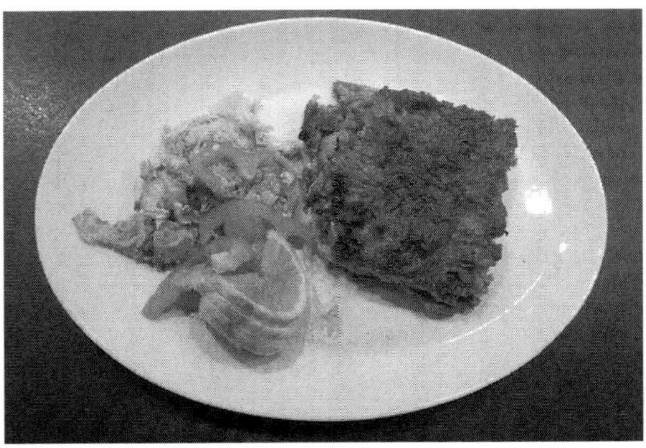

Ingredients:

1. 4 pounds fresh chicken meat.
2. ½ cup of unsalted butter.
3. 6 minced garlic cloves.
4. 2 cups of chicken broth.
5. 2 cups of lemon juice.
6. 1 cup of nicely grated parmesan cheese.
7. 1 tbsp paprika and 1 teaspoon thyme.
8. Salt and pepper to taste.

Instruction:

1. Preheat oven to 190^{oc}.
2. Place chicken meat in a bowl and season with paprika, pepper, and salt.
3. Pour half of unsalted butter into frying pan and melt over medium heat. Add chicken and sauté for 4-6 minutes.
4. Pour remaining butter in a large frying pan and melt over medium heat. Add garlic and fry for 2-3 minutes.
5. Add chicken broth, parmesan cheese, lemon juice thyme to garlic pan and stir will its cooks.
6. Add chicken meat and cook for 20-25 minutes.

7. Serve as desired.

Chicken Bacon Burgers

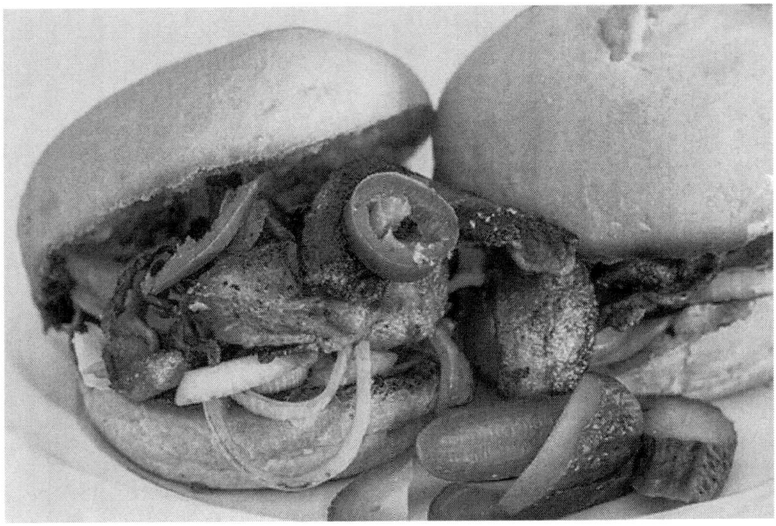

Ingredients:

1. 4 pounds fresh shredded chicken meat.
2. 2 pounds shredded bacon.
3. 6 toasted hamburger buns.
4. 2 large eggs. Beaten.
5. 2 cups fresh breadcrumb.
6. 2 well minced onion.
7. 4 tbsp olive oil.
8. 1 cup egg mayonnaise.

9. 1 tbsp curry paste.
10. 3 finely chopped lettuce leaves.
11. Salt and pepper to taste.

Instruction:

1. Place beaten egg, onion, breadcrumb, shredded chicken in a bowl and mix well. Add pepper and 1 teaspoon of salt and blend to form chicken patties. Divide patty as desired and set patties aside in a plate.
2. Mix mayonnaise and curry paste in a small bowl and set aside
3. Over medium heat, fry bacon in frying pan until slightly brown. Set aside to drain.
4. Pour oil into pan and heat over medium heat. Add chicken patties and fry for 8-10 minutes until brown.
5. Divide lettuce into bacon bun and top each bun with bacon, chicken patties and curried mayonnaise.

Paprika Chicken

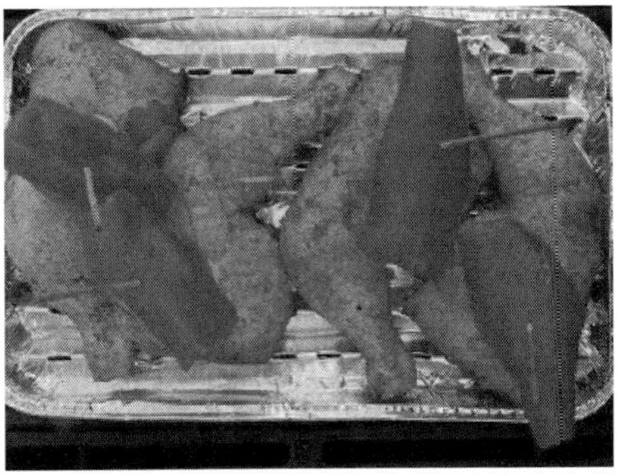

Ingredients:

1. 4 pounds fresh chicken meat.
2. 2 full tbsp paprika.
3. 4 finely minced garlic cloves.
4. 2 medium size chopped onion
5. 4 large finely sliced tomatoes.
6. 1 cup fresh finely minced parsley.
7. 1 cup chicken broth.
8. 2 tbsp olive oil.
9. 1 tbsp pepper and 2 tsp salt to season.

Instruction:

1. Over medium heat, heat the oil in a frying pan.
2. Place chicken in a bowl and season with salt and pepper. Fry chicken in oil for 6-8 minutes until golden. Place on a tray with paper towel and allow oil to drain.
3. Place pan with oil back over medium heat and add stir-fry onion and garlic for 2 minutes.
4. Add paprika and tomato and stir-fry for 1 minute. Add chicken broth and chicken meat and cook for 15-20 minutes.
5. Reduce heat and allow to simmer.
6. Serve as desired with fresh parsley leaves on top.

Stuffed Chicken Breast

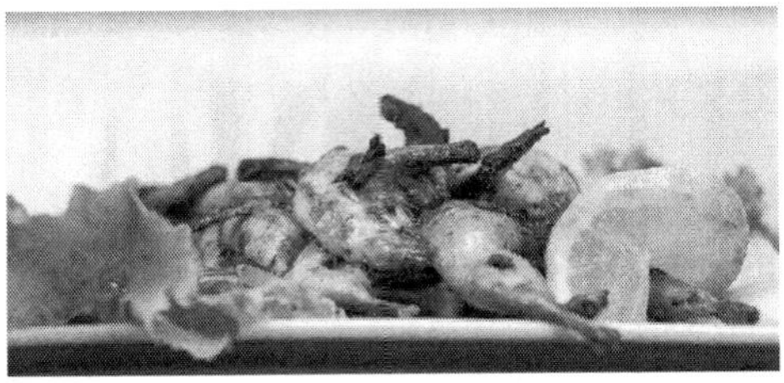

Ingredients:

1. 2 pounds pounded boneless chicken breast.
2. 2 packaged fresh green spinach leaves.
3. 2 diced apple.
4. 1 cup of minced cheese.
5. ½ cup sour cream.
6. 6 finely minced garlic cloves.
7. 2 tbsp parsley.
8. 2 tbsp pepper and salt to taste.

Instruction:

1. Preheat oven to 185^{oc}.
2. Place spinach in a bowl and microwave for 4 minutes.
3. Pour cheese, cream, apple, and garlic in a bowl. Add spinach and soak thoroughly.
4. Place pounded flattened chicken on a baking tray. Divide into equal halves and insert spinach-cheese mixture and parsley leaves into each and roll up tightly for baking.
5. Bake in preheated oven for 30-40 minutes until golden.

Coconut Chicken

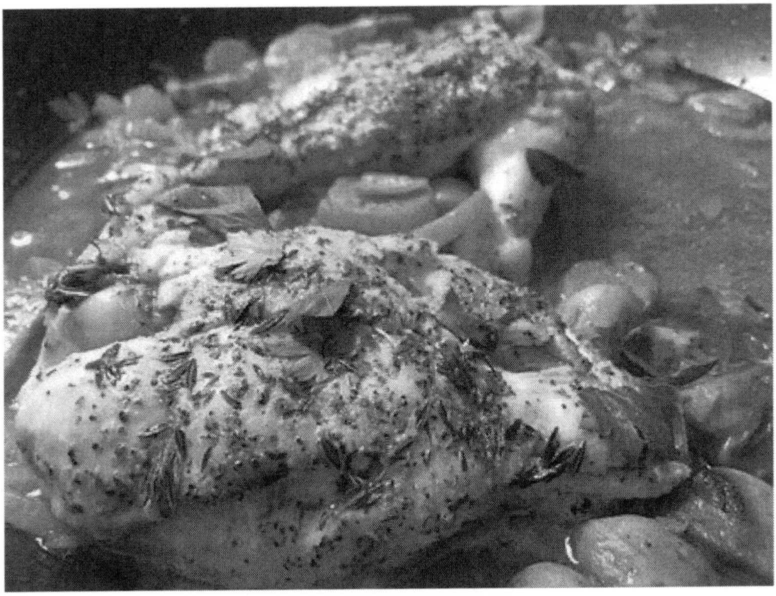

Ingredients:

1. 4 pounds boneless chicken breast.
2. 2 medium can coconut milk.
3. 1 large fresh diced coconut head.
4. 4 shredded garlic cloves.
5. 2 tbsp curry powder.
6. 3 tbsp vegetable oil.

7. 1 finely minced onion.
8. 2 sachet tomato paste.
9. Salt and pepper to taste.

Instruction:

1. Coat chicken breast with pepper and salt seasoning.
2. In a deep frying pan, heat oil and stir-fry curry powder for 2 minutes.
3. Add diced coconut, onion and garlic and stir-fry for 2 minutes. Then coat seasoned chicken with curry oil mixture and cook for 8-10 minutes over medium heat.

4. Reduce heat to simmer. Add tomato paste, coconut milk, pepper, and stir. Allow cooking for 35-40 minutes (Stir occasionally).

Turkey Meatloaf

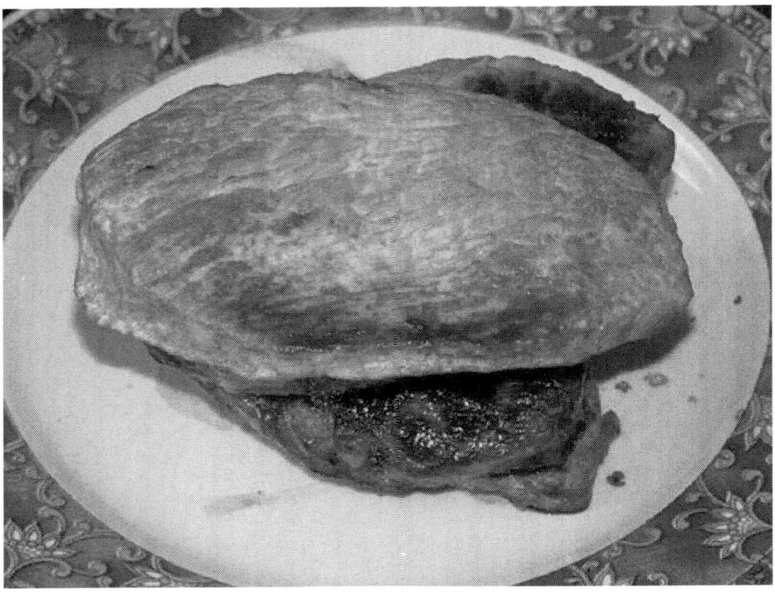

Ingredients:

1. 3 pounds fresh shredded turkey meat.

2. 2 cup breadcrumb.
3. 3 tbsp butter.
4. 1 large finely chopped onion.
5. 4 minced garlic cloves.
6. 2 large eggs.
7. 3 tbsp Worcestershire sauce.
8. 1 tbsp black pepper.
9. 1 tsp salt.

Instruction:

1. Preheat oven to 180^{oc}.
2. Pour butter in a frying pan and let it melt.
3. Stir-fry onion and garlic in melted butter for 4 minutes.

4. Add Worcestershire sauce, eggs, breadcrumbs and turkey meat to melted butter pan. Blend.
5. Fetch meatloaf mixture and insert into baking loaf pan of desired shape and size.
6. Place into oven and bake for 50-60 minutes until golden brown.
7. Remove from oven and let it cool then serve immediately.

Turkey Rissoles

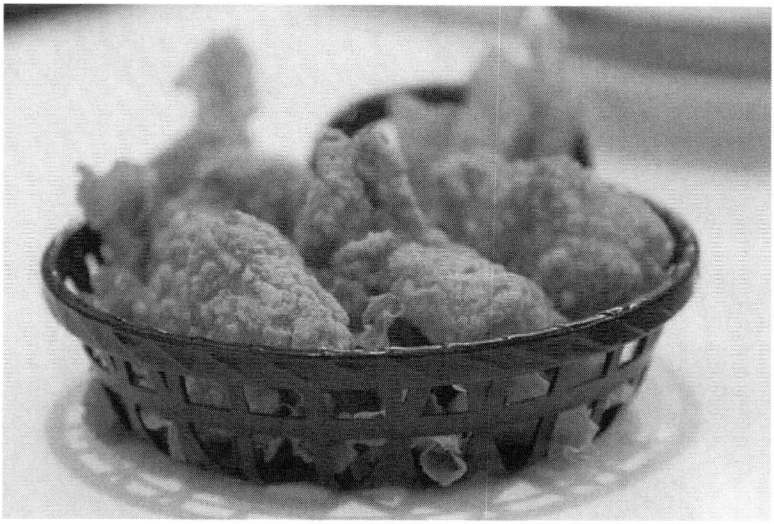

Ingredients:

1. 4 pounds shredded turkey meat.
2. 2 large eggs.
3. 2 tbsp olive oil.
4. 4 minced garlic cloves.
5. 1 large finely chopped onion.
6. 3 tbsp fresh parsley leaves.
7. 1 tbsp pepper powder.

8. Salt.

Instruction:

1. Place turkey in a large bowl and season with pepper and salt.
2. Add egg, onion, garlic, parsley, and process in a food processor over medium-high heat till mixture combines well.
3. Roll mixture into patties to form rissoles for frying.
4. Pour olive oil into frying pan to heat then fry rissoles for 6-8 minutes until it turns golden.
5. Allow cooling then serve immediately.

Part 11

CHAPTER SIXTEEN

KETO MEATS

Meats are also essential meals to be consumed during a keto dieting program. Meats from animals are recommended like beef, bacon (pork), turkey, fish or any other edible animal flesh. This is because meats are good suppliers of fat and oil. Here is a quick recipe for mouth-watering keto meat diet accompanied by creamy pesto sauce.

Nut Stuffed Pork Chops

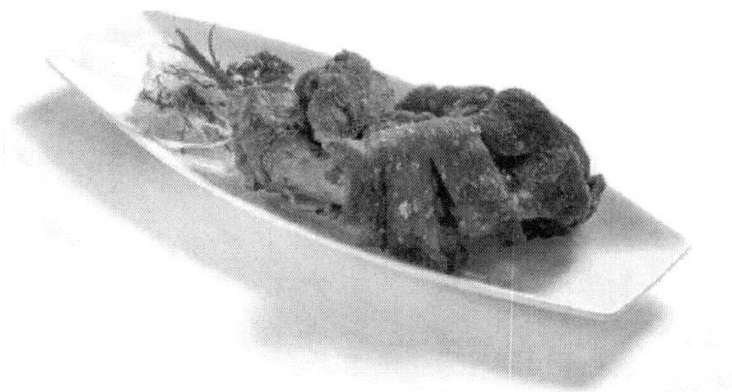

Ingredients:

1. 8 thick pork chops with stuffing pocket.
2. 1 cup diced apple.
3. 3 cups breadcrumb.
4. 1 cup minced cheddar cheese.
5. $1^1/_2$ cup lemon juice.
6. 3 tbsp finely shredded toasted pecans nut.
7. 3 tbsp melted butter.
8. Salt and pepper to taste.

Instruction:

1. Preheat oven to 190^{oc}.
2. Season chops with pepper and salt.
3. Pour melted butter into a large bowl. Add 2 cups breadcrumb, cheese, apple, 1 cup lemon juice. Blend until well mixed.
4. Stuff each chops with mixture. Deep each in remaining lemon juice and coat with remaining breadcrumbs.
5. Place chops in the baking pan, cover and bake for 16-20 minutes at medium-high heat.
6. Reduce heat and uncover. Bake on for 25- 30 minutes until golden.
7. Allow to cool and ser immediately.

Roasted Keto Pork Sauced with Loin Grainy Mustard

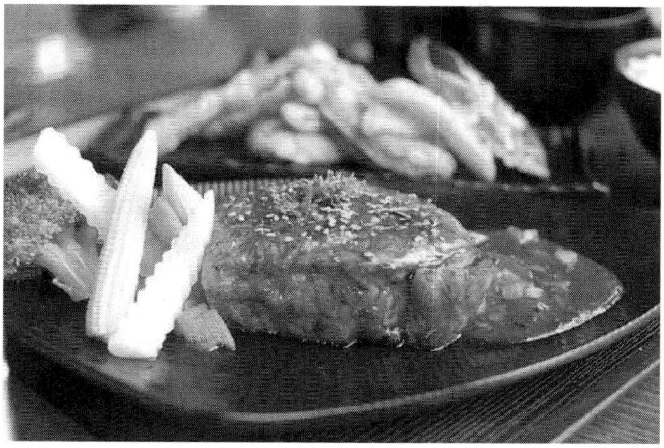

Ingredients:

1. 2 pounds fresh pork loin fillet.
2. 2 tbsp wholegrain mustard.
3. 2 tbsp unsalted butter.
4. 2 tbsp olive oil.
5. 1 cup pork or chicken broth.
6. 2 tsp flour.

7. 1 tsp black pepper powder.
8. ½ tsp salt.

Instruction:

1. Place pork on a tray and flatten then season pork with a sprinkle of salt and pepper.
2. Pour oil into large frying pan and heat. Add pork and cook for 4 minutes until done then cover and set aside.
3. In another smaller frying pan, add butter, flour, wholegrain mustard to pan over medium heat and keep stirring until butter melts. Add broth, little more salt and pepper and let it cook till the mixture becomes thick.
4. Serve pork loin with grainy mustard sauce.

Keto Lamb Chops with Kalamata Tapenade

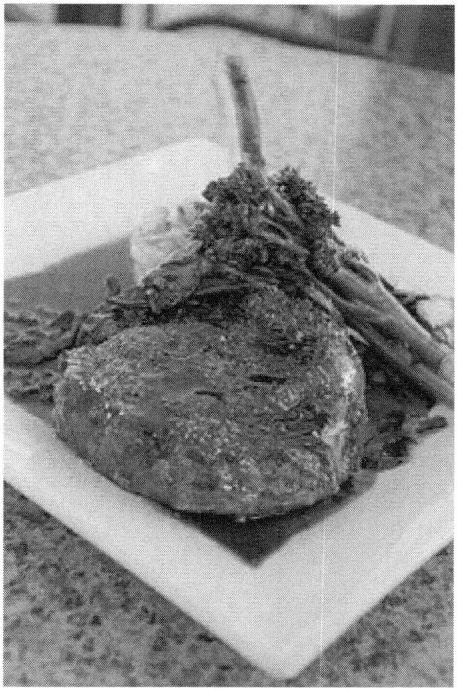

Ingredients:

1. 3 pounds lamb loin chops.
2. 2 cups Kalamata olive.
3. 2 tbsp fresh lemon juice and 1 tbsp sherry.
4. 2 tbsp olive oil.
5. 2 tsp salted anchovies.

6. 4 tbsp finely minced capers.
7. 1 tbsp paprika and cumin powder.
8. 5 finely minced garlic cloves.
9. 1 tsp salt and 1 tbsp pepper to taste.

Instruction:

1. To prepare tapenade olive paste: Place kalamata olives, anchovies, capers and puree in food processor. Add olive oil, lemon juice, sherry, garlic, pepper, salt, and process until well mixed then set aside.
2. Pour olive oil in a pan. Add cumin, paprika, pepper, salt, and blend.
3. Coat lamb chops with cumin mixture and then stir-cook over low heat for 5 minutes. Then increase heat and let it cook until done and thick.
4. Serve chops on plate and top with tapenade olive paste sauce.

Rosemary-Garlic Lamb Racks

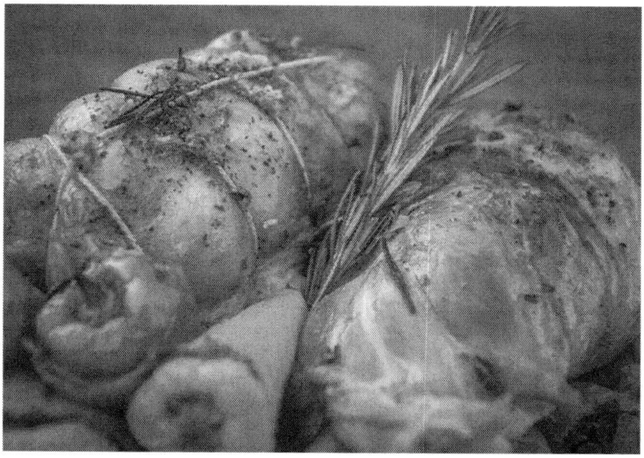

Ingredients:

1. 6 lamb racks.
2. 4 minced garlic cloves.
3. 4 fresh sprigs rosemary leaves. Sliced.
4. 2 tbsp fresh honey.
5. 3 tbsp mustard grain.
6. 3 tbsp mint sauce.
7. Salt and pepper to taste.

Instruction:

1. Preheat oven to 190^{oc}.
2. Place lamb racks o a plate and remove excess fat.

3. Carefully cut each lamb rack at the top to create an opening. Carefully insert garlic and rosemary into the openings.
4. Place honey, mint sauce, and mustard grain in a bowl and mix together.
5. Coat each lamb rack with honey mixture and allow to soak in the mixture for 15 minutes.
6. Remove lamb racks and place in a baking dish. Bake for 20-25 minutes until done.
7. Allow to cool and serve as desired.

Lamb Leg with Dried Tomato Pesto

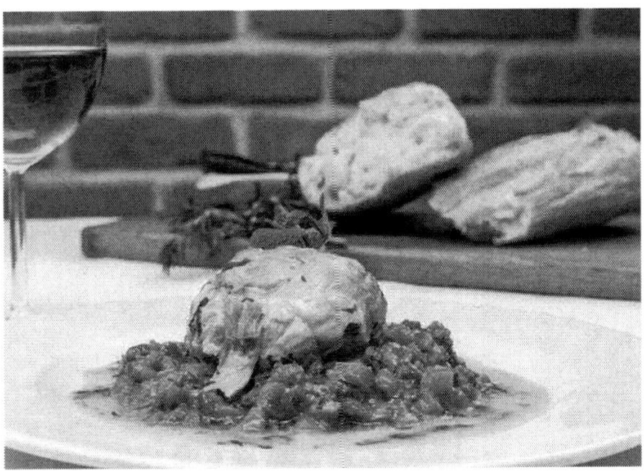

Ingredients:

1. 3 pounds boneless lamb leg.

2. 4 large sundried tomatoes. Sliced.
3. 4 finely minced garlic cloves.
4. 3 tbsp fresh basil pesto.
5. 1 cup grated lemon juice.
6. 1 tsp mustard.
7. 1 tbsp olive oil and butter.
8. 2 tbsp vinegar.
9. 1 cup breadcrumb.
10. Salt and pepper to taste.

Instruction:

1. Preheat oven to 180^{oc}.
2. Place tomato, basil pesto, garlic and lemon juice in a bowl and mix. Add breadcrumb and mix together until well mixed to form a dough.
3. Divide lamb leg into medium parts and create an opening with a knife and insert little mixture into opening. Heat olive oil and butter in pan and cook lamb till brownish. Then set aside.
4. Season with salt and pepper then sprinkle vinegar and mustard all over lamb. Then place in oven and roast for 60 minutes. Cover and set aside.

5. Add a little water to tomato and basil pesto mixture and cook for 6-8 minutes over medium heat to make pesto sauce.
6. Serve lamb with basil pesto sauce.

Sirloin with Blue Cheese Compound Butter

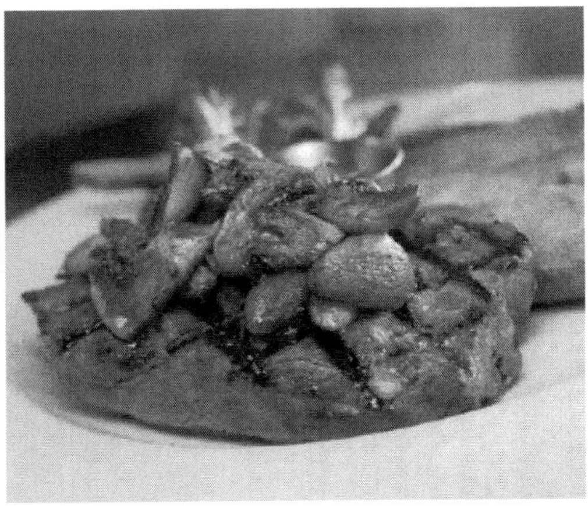

Ingredients:

1. 2 pounds sirloin steaks.
2. 1 cup of crumbled blue cheese.
3. ½ cup unsalted compound butter.
4. 3 finely minced garlic clove.
5. 2 tbsp finely minced chive/rosemary leaves.
6. 2 tbsp olive oil.
7. 1 tbsp black pepper powder.

8. 1 tsp salt.

Instruction:

1. Place blue cheese, butter, rosemary/chives, garlic, pepper, salt in a bowl and mix thoroughly.
2. Roll mixture into a square and cover tightly. Then refrigerate for 1:40 minutes or more.
3. Place sirloin steaks on a tray and season with salt and pepper.
4. Pour oil into pan and heat. Add sirloin and grill for 8-10 minutes until slightly brownish.
5. Serve sirloin on plates and top with butter mixture.

Garlic-Braised Short Ribs

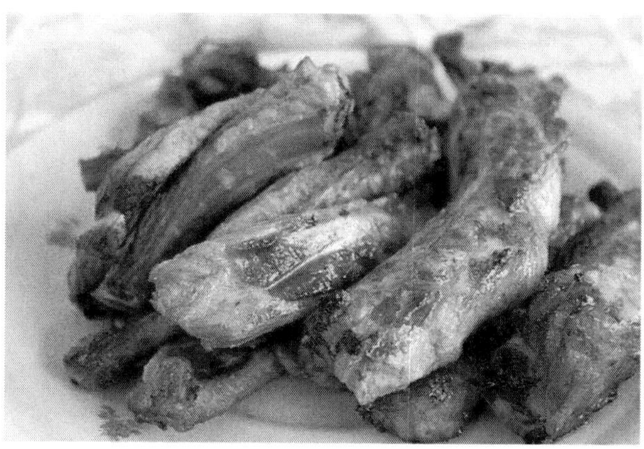

Ingredients:

1. 4 pounds beef short ribs.
2. 12 finely minced garlic cloves.
3. 4 tbsp unsalted butter.
4. 2 tbsp finely minced rosemary leaves.
5. 1 large finely diced onion.
6. $1^1/_2$ cup chicken broth.
7. 3 tbsp olive oil.
8. 1 cup white wine.
9. Salt and black pepper to taste.

Instruction:

1. Preheat oven to 190^{oc}.
2. Place beef short ribs on a tray and season all over with salt and pepper.
3. Heat olive oil in a pan and cook short ribs for 8-10 minutes until light brown. Remove ribs and set aside then lightly fry garlic and onion in same oil.
4. Pour chicken broth and wine into the pan. Add rosemary and short ribs, stir and allow to braise over medium-low heat for 1:30 minutes or more. Stir occasionally for even cooking.

5. Add butter and more garlic to braising short ribs until done.
6. Serve in plates immediately.

Bacon-Wrapped Beef Tenderloin

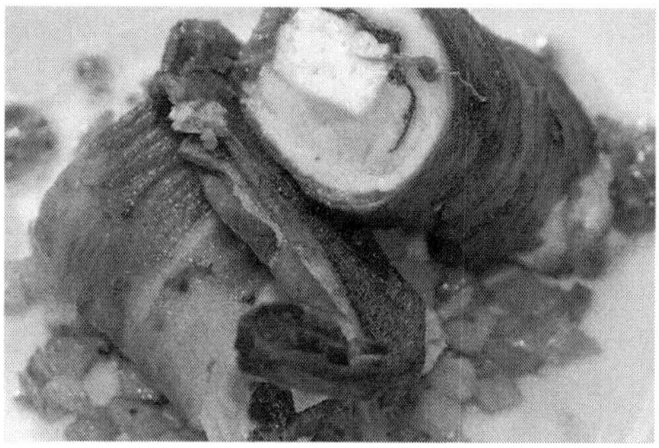

Ingredients:

1. 4 pounds beef tenderloin. Sliced.
2. 1 pounds smoked bacon. Sliced.
3. ½ cup shredded unsalted butter.
4. ½ cup canola oil.
5. 4 finely minced garlic cloves.
6. 1 large minced onion.
7. ½ cup peppercorn.
8. 1 cup beef broth.
9. ½ cup fresh whiskey.
10. 2 tbsp black pepper.

11. Salt to taste.

Instruction:

1. Preheat oven to 190ºC.
2. Place bacon and tenderloin in a bowl and season with salt and pepper.
3. Place on a plastic wrap and roll-up tightly at both ends then refrigerate for an hour until bacon and beef stick together.
4. Pour canola oil into the pan to heat. Remove beef-bacon mixture and fry for 6-8 minutes until golden brown.
5. Insert into oven and roast for 25-30 minutes. Then cover and set aside.
6. Pour a little oil in a pan and fry garlic and onion. Reduce heat then add peppercorn and whiskey to prepare peppercorn sauce.
7. Increase heat and add beef broth and butter. Add salt and pepper then simmer.
8. Serve bacon slices with peppercorn sauce.

Cheeseburger Casserole

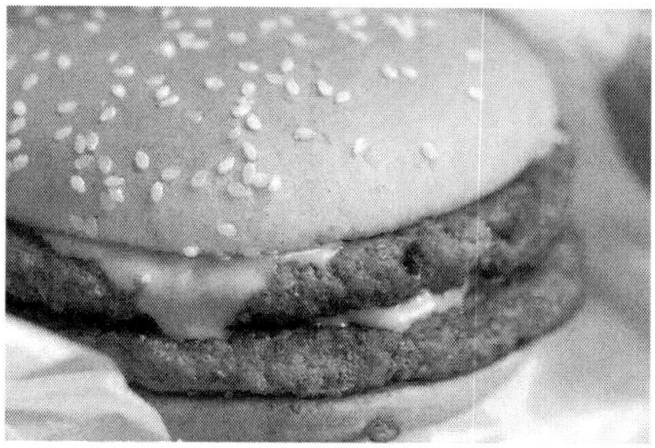

Ingredients:

1. 4 pounds lean ground beef.
2. 2 cup shredded cheese.
3. 1 large finely minced onion.
4. 4 tbsp flour.
5. 4 fresh finely sliced tomatoes.
6. 1 cup ketchup.
7. 2 tbsp fresh mustard.
8. 1 tbsp black pepper powder.

Instruction:

1. Preheat oven to 190^{oc}.
2. Heat oil in a pan then add beef, onion, pepper, salt and cook for 6-8 minutes. Stir occasionally
3. Sprinkle flour over beef in pan and stir. Add mustard, ketchup, tomatoes and stir till well mix.

4. Place beef mixture in baking dish then sprinkles cheese over mixture. Bake in the oven for 20 minutes.
5. Set aside to cool and serve immediately.

Italian Beef Burger

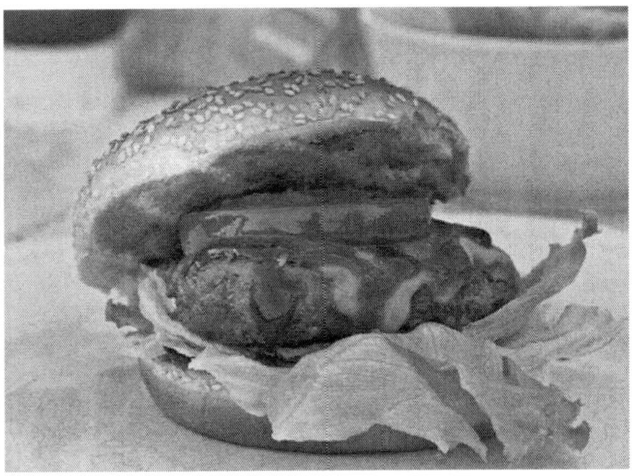

Ingredients:

1. 2 pounds ground beef.
2. 1 tbsp Italian seasoning.
3. 1 tbsp garlic powder.
4. 4 tbsp Worcestershire sauce.
5. 4 tbsp butter.

6. 4 tbsp cheese.
7. 4 tbsp olive oil.
8. 5 finely minced garlic cloves.
9. 1 large finely minced onion.
10. 2 tbsp finely minced parsley.
11. 4 cups beef broth.
12. 1 tbsp black pepper.
13. 2 tsp salt.

Instruction:

1. Preheat oven to 200^{oc}.
2. Melt butter in the pan then add pepper, garlic, onion, Italian seasoning and cook for 10-12 minutes.
3. Over medium heat add beef broth, Worcestershire sauce, parsley, and simmer.

4. In a large bowl, add beef, pepper, Worcestershire sauce, cheese, Italian seasoning and mix well until it forms thick patties then form burger patties into desired size and shape.
5. Place burger on buns and grill for 8-10 minutes. Add pepper butter mixture over top of burger and grill for 4 minutes.
6. Serve immediately as desired.

Part 12

CHAPTER SEVENTEEN

KETO DESSERTS

Desserts are sweet course eaten at the end of the main meal. A typical dessert course usually consists of sweet food, snacks and beverages like a dessert wine, liqueur, nuts, coffee and other foods of savory. Desserts aid in the smooth and easy digestion of meals. Be sure to consume a mouthwatering dessert to conclude your keto meals.

Pumpkin Spiced Fat Bombs

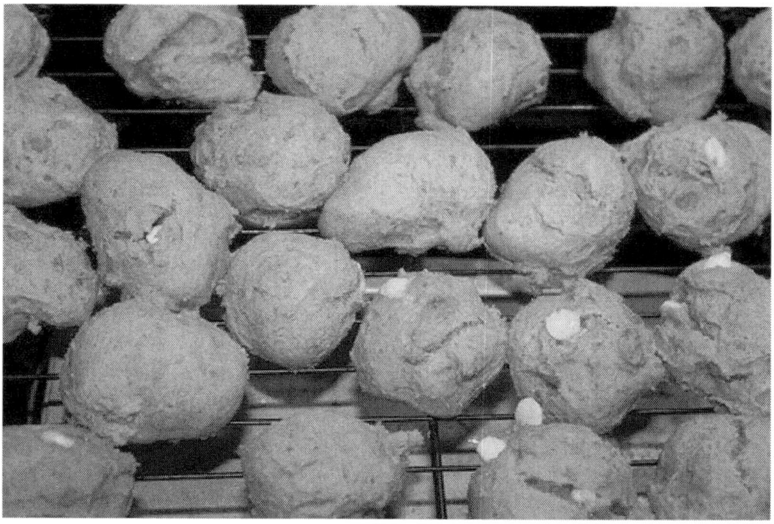

Ingredients:

1. 2 cup pumpkin puree.
2. 1 cup coconut oil.
3. 2 tsp nutmeg.
4. 1 tbsp cinnamon.
5. 1 tbsp stevia to taste.

Instruction:

1. Pour pumpkin puree in a large bowl.

2. Add nutmeg, coconut oil, cinnamon, stevia, and blend.
3. Refrigerate in the freezer for 40 minutes. Remove and roll into fat bombs.
4. Put fat bombs into the refrigerator for 1 hour.
5. Serve immediately or store in the freezer.

Creamy Banana Fat Bombs

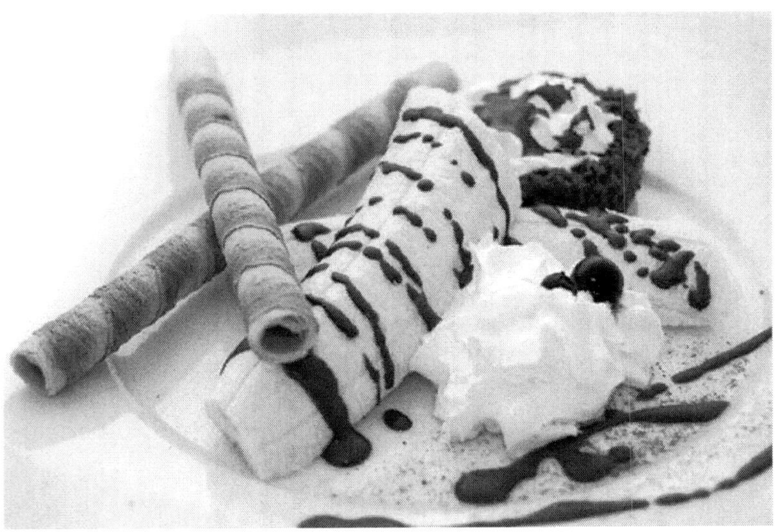

Ingredients:

1. 6 pureed bananas.
2. 1 cup cream cheese.
3. ½ cup butter.
4. ½ cup cocoa powder.
5. 1 tbsp stevia.

Instruction:

1. Pour banana puree in a pot over medium-high heat.
2. Add butter, cocoa powder, stevia and allow to boil for 6-8 minutes until thick.
3. Pour content into cups and allow to cool then top with cream cheese.
4. Serve immediately or refrigerate.

Blueberry Fat Bombs

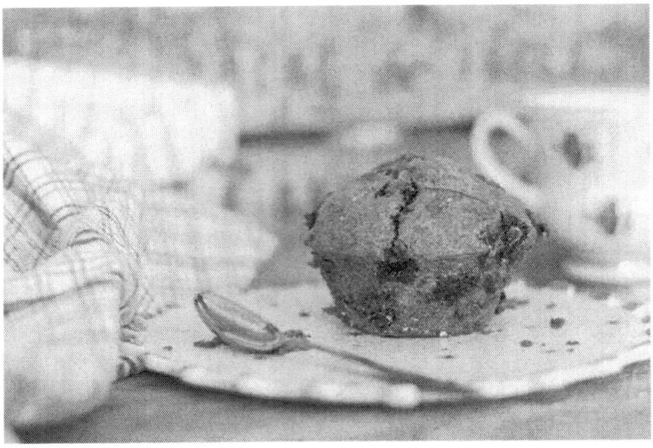

Ingredients:

1. 6 cup blueberry.
2. ½ cup coconut oil.
3. ½ cup butter.
4. ½ cup cream cheese.
5. 2 tbsp stevia.

Instruction:

1. Pour blueberry puree in a blender. Add cream cheese and coconut cream and blend until smooth.
2. Melt butter and coconut oil over medium-low heat in a pan. Set aside to cool.
3. Pour into blender with blueberry mixture and blend. Add stevia and blend until thick and smooth.
4. Pout pureed blueberry mixture into small cups or containers and refrigerated in the freezer for 1 hour or more.
5. Remove and enjoy immediately.

Spiced Chocolate Fat Bombs

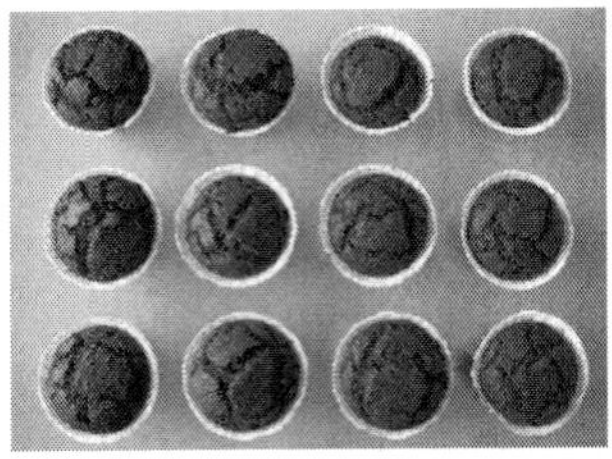

Ingredients:

1. 2 cup coconut milk.
2. ½ cup cocoa powder.
3. 2 tbsp vanilla extract.
4. 2 tbsp chocolate extract.
5. 1 tbsp cinnamon.
6. 2 tsp ground paprika.
7. 1 tbsp stevia extract.

Instruction:

1. Pour coconut milk in a bowl.
2. Add all other ingredients/sweeteners and blend until well combined.
3. Pour mixture into small cups or ice-cubes and refrigerate in the freezer for 1 hour or more until thick.
4. Remove and enjoy immediately.

Chocolate-Coconut Treats

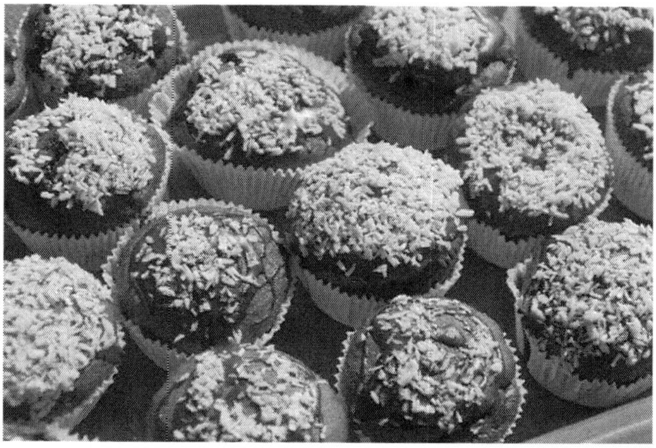

Ingredients:

1. 2 cup coconut milk.
2. 1 cup cocoa powder.
3. ½ cup dried coconut.
4. 1 pack milk biscuit. Crushed.
5. 1 tbsp chocolate extract.
6. 2 tsp stevia extract.

Instruction:

1. Place crushed biscuits in a bowl.
2. Add coconut milk and other ingredients and blend until well combined.
3. Pour mixture into cups and refrigerate for 40 minutes.
4. Remove and enjoy immediately.

Almond Butter Fudge

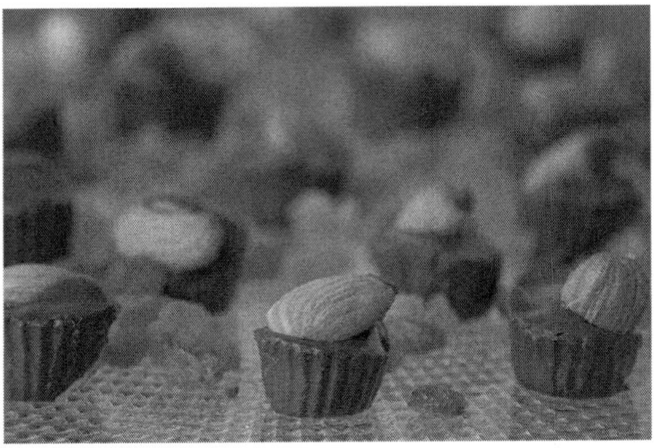

Ingredients:

1. 1 cup almond butter.
2. ½ cup pure honey.
3. 1 cup cocoa powder.
4. 1 cup melted coconut oil.
5. 1 tsp vanilla extract.
6. ½ tsp stevia extract.

Instruction:

1. Pour coconut oil and honey in a bowl. Blend.
2. Add almond butter, cocoa powder, vanilla extract, stevia extract and blend until smooth like a puree.

3. Pour mixture into small cups or cake muffins and refrigerate for 40 minutes or more.
4. Serve and enjoy immediately.

Nutty Shortbread Cookies

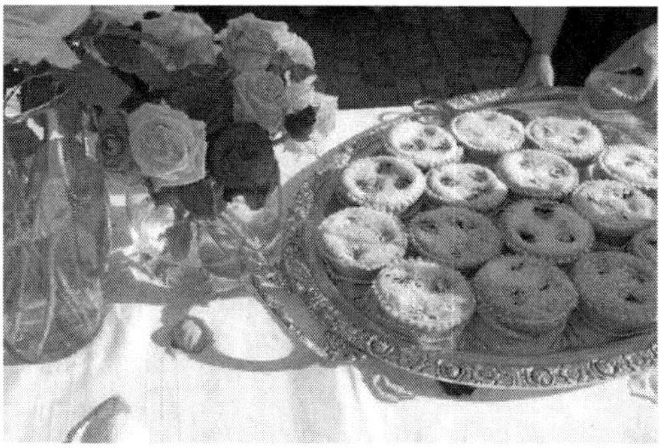

Ingredients:

1. 1 cup nicely chopped coconut.
2. 2 cup flour.
3. 1 cup milk.
4. ½ cup unsalted soft butter.
5. 1 tsp vanilla extract.
6. 4 tbsp sugar.
7. Salt to taste.

Instruction:

1. Preheat oven to 190^{oc}.
2. Pour flour into a bowl. Add milk, butter, sugar, vanilla extract, and mix well to form a dough.
3. Add chopped coconut pieces and mix well with dough. Shape into small dough balls and put into baking dish.
4. Bake in preheated oven for 30 minutes.
5. Serve immediately or store in a flask.

Vanilla-Almond Ice Pops

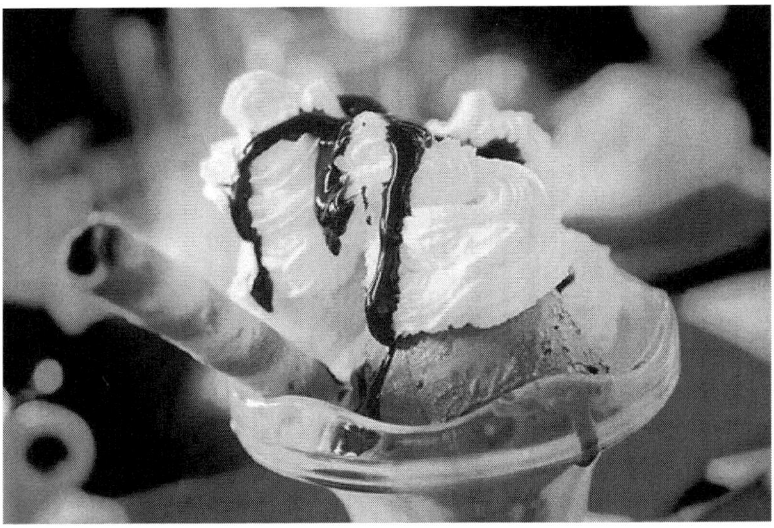

Ingredients:

1. 2 cup unsweetened almond milk.

2. 1 cup chopped almond nut.
3. 1 tbsp vanilla extract.
4. 2 tbsp honey.
5. 2 tbsp sugar.

Instruction:

1. Pour almond milk into a bowl.
2. Add almond nut pieces, vanilla extract, honey, sugar and blend until smooth.
3. Pour mixture into ice popsicles and refrigerate in the freezer for 50-60 minute.
4. Enjoy immediately.

Raspberry Cheesecake

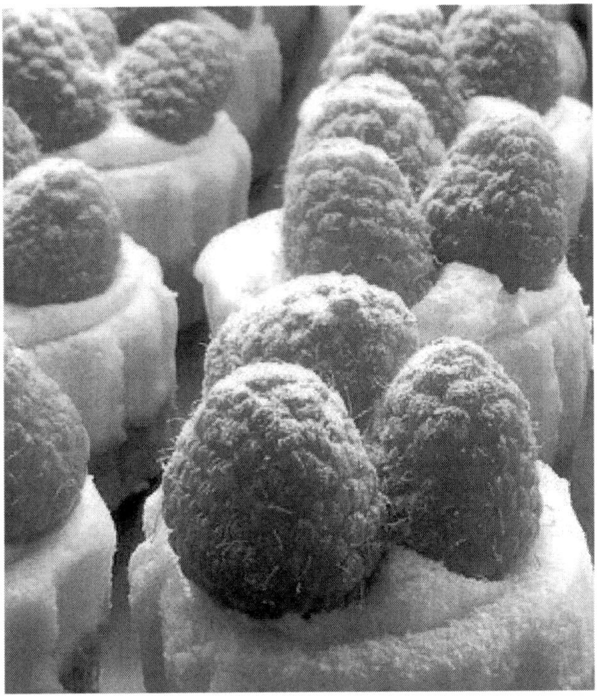

Ingredients:

1. 1 cup fresh raspberry.
2. ½ cup unsalted butter.
3. 1 cup cream cheese.
4. 1 tin condensed liquid milk.
5. ½ cup lemon juice.
6. 2 large pack plain biscuits. Crushed.
7. 2 gelatin sheet.
8. ½ tsp vanilla extract.

Instruction:

1. Melt butter and pour into a bowl. Add crushed biscuit crumb and blend until thick and smooth. Carefully pour mixture into a medium size cake tin and spread evenly then refrigerate for 20 minutes.
2. Pour cream cheese in another bowl. Add milk, lemon juice, vanilla extract and blend. Set aside.
3. Puree half cup of raspberry and set aside the rest.
4. Dissolve gelatin with 4 tbsp of water. Pour half in cream cheese mixture and a half in raspberry puree.
5. Add raspberry puree to cream cheese mixture and stir in a swirling manner.
6. Remove cake tin with biscuit crumb and then pour cream cheese mixture inside.
7. Drop remaining raspberry on top of the cheesecake, cover tightly and refrigerate for 10-12 hours.

Peanut Butter Mousse

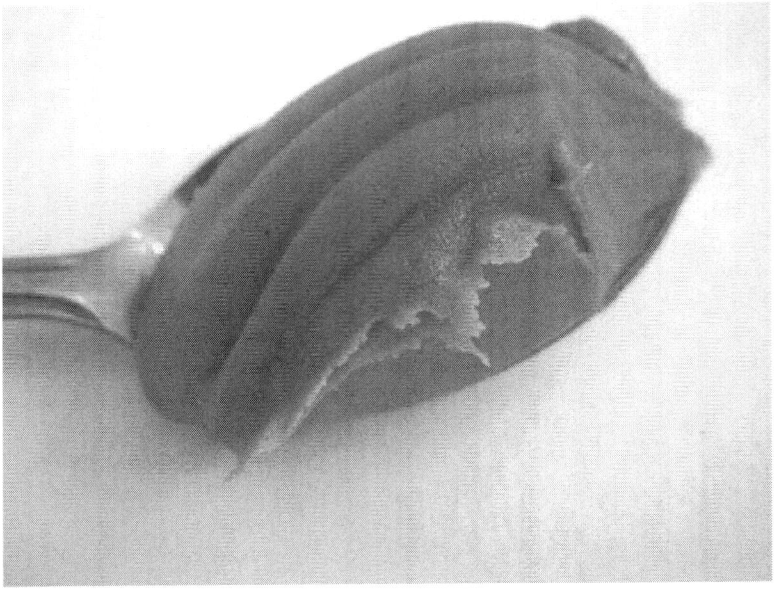

Ingredients:

1. 2 cup peanut butter.
2. ½ cup crushed peanut.
3. 1 cup heavy cream.
4. 1 cup cream cheese.
5. ½ cup milk.
6. 2 beaten eggs.
7. 1 tsp vanilla extract.
8. 1 tsp stevia extract.

Instruction:

1. Pour heavy cream and cream cheese in a bowl and mix.
2. Add peanut butter, vanilla extract, stevia, beaten egg and mix well until thick and smooth.
3. Refrigerate mixture for 30 minutes.
4. Serve in cups and top with crushed peanuts.

Part 13

CHAPTER EIGHTEEN

STAPLES

Staples are basic foods and ingredients for dieting. Keto staples come in a wide range and variety. It depends on your choice of staples. Here are recipes for keto staples.

Avocado-Herb Compound Butter

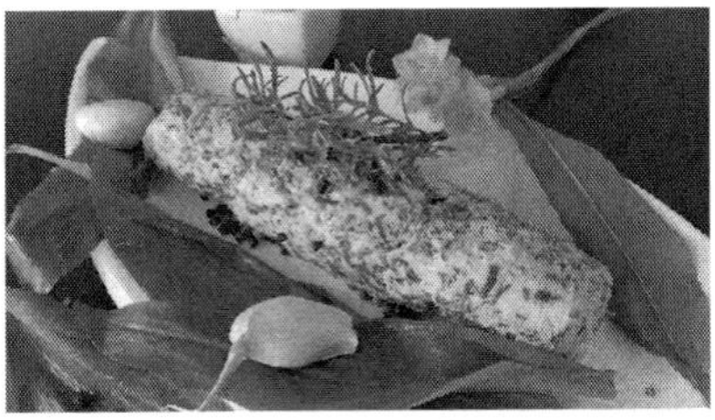

Ingredients:

1. 4 avocados.
2. 1 cup soft unsalted butter.
3. 4 tbsp finely minced parsley.
4. 2 tbsp finely minced cilantro leaves.
5. 2 large finely minced garlic cloves.
6. 2 tsp ground cumin.
7. 4 tbsp lemon juice.
8. Salt and ground black pepper to taste.

Instruction:

1. Melt butter and pour into a bowl.
2. Divide avocados, remove flesh and put in a bowl with butter. Stir until good mix.
3. Add lemon juice, parsley, cilantro, cumin, garlic and blend until good mix and thick.
4. Pour mixture into small cake muffins and refrigerate for 5 hours.

5. Serve and enjoy immediately.

Strawberry Butter

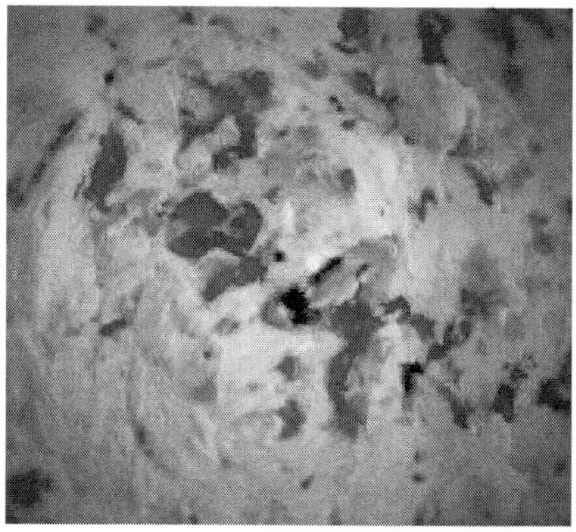

Ingredients:

1. 2 cup fresh diced strawberry.
2. ½ cup unsalted butter.
3. ½ cup fresh cream.
4. ½ tsp vanilla extract.
5. 1 tsp stevia extract or any sweetener of choice.

Instruction:

1. Melt butter and pour into a bowl. Add cream and blend.

2. Puree 1 cup of diced strawberry and pour in bowl with butter. Blend until good mix.
3. Add vanilla extract and stevia. Blend until good mix.
4. Pour mixture into cups or cake muffin and refrigerate for 4 hours.
5. Serve and enjoy immediately.

Herb Balsamic Dressing

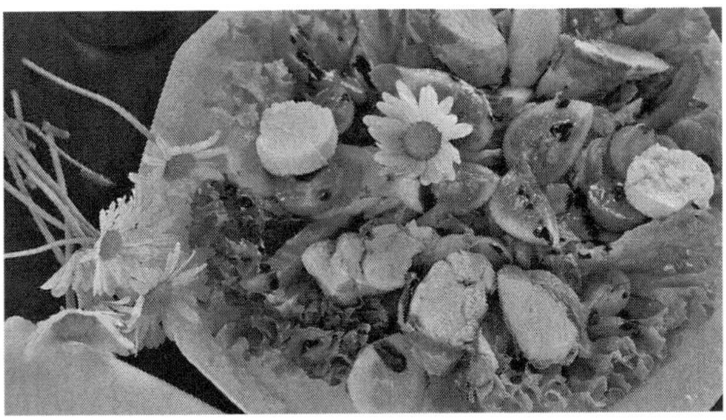

Ingredients:

1. 1 cup fresh Italian balsamic vinegar.
2. 1 cup canola oil.
3. 4 tbsp fresh honey.
4. 4 tbsp finely minced chive.
5. 2 tbsp finely minced parsley.

6. 2 tbsp finely minced basil.
7. ½ tsp salt.

Instruction:

1. Pour vinegar into a bowl. Add honey, canola oil, salt and stir until well mixed.
2. Add chive, parsley, basil and stir to mix.
3. Pour mixture into cups or muffins and refrigerate for 5 hours.
4. Serve and enjoy immediately.

Herb Keto Kale Pesto

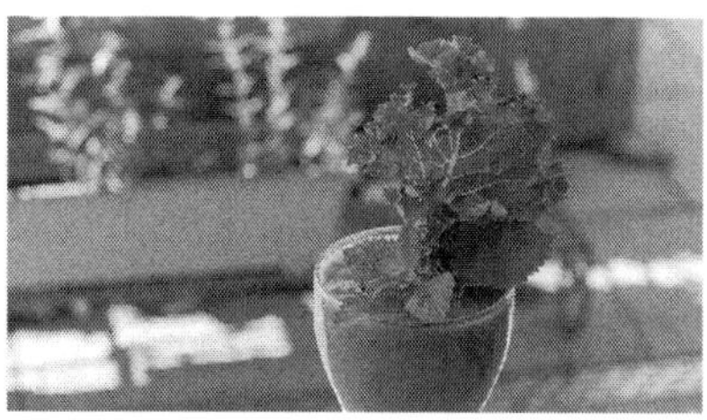

Ingredients:

1. 2 pounds fresh finely minced kale cabbage with stems cut-off.
2. 1 cup parmesan cheese.

3. ½ cup extra virgin olive oil.
4. ½ cup minced chive.
5. ½ cup minced parsley.
6. ½ cup minced basil.
7. 4 large minced garlic cloves.
8. Salt and ground pepper to taste.

Instruction:

1. Place kale, chive, parsley, basil, garlic in a food processor.
2. Add olive oil, cheese, salt, pepper and blend in food processor until well mixed.
3. Serve immediately.

Keto Hollandaise

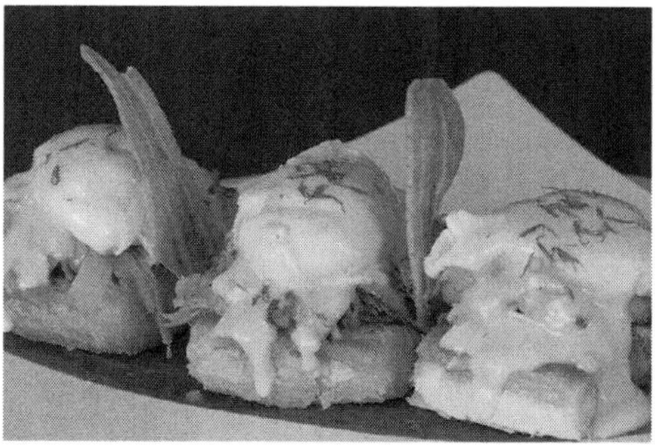

Ingredients:

1. 2 cup unsalted butter.
2. 6 egg yolks.
3. 1 cup Parmesan cheese.
4. 1 cup vinegar.
5. ½ cup minced parsley.
6. Salt and ground pepper.

Instruction:

1. Melt butter in a pan.
2. Pour egg yolk and cheese in a bowl and whisk well. Add vinegar, parsley, salt, pepper and whisk well.
3. Pour egg yolk mixture into the pan with butter, whisk and stir-cook over low simmering heat until

thick. If it becomes too thick, add little hot water and simmer again.

4. Serve hollandaise sauce and enjoy with rice or beans.

Keto Green Basil Dressing

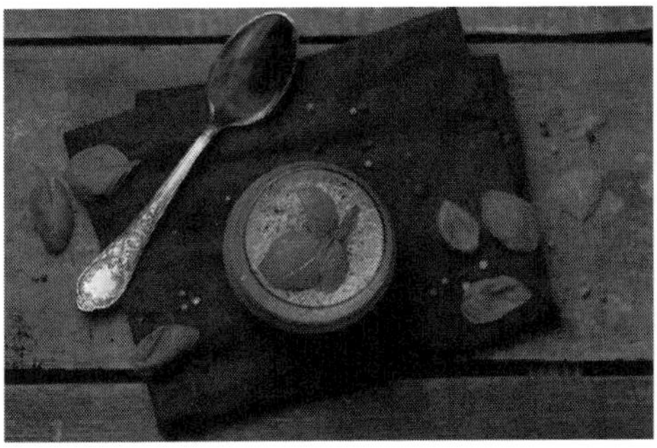

Ingredients:

1. 1 cup sour cream.
2. 1 cup mayonnaise.
3. ½ cup lemon juice.
4. 1 cup chopped basil.
5. 2 tbsp chopped chive.
6. 4 finely minced garlic cloves.
7. 2 minced scallions.
8. ½ cup cooked halibut fillet.
9. Salt and ground pepper to taste.

Instruction:

1. Prepare all ingredients and put in a food processor.
2. Add a little water and blend until thick and smooth.
3. Serve in cups and enjoy.

Keto Creamy Mayonnaise

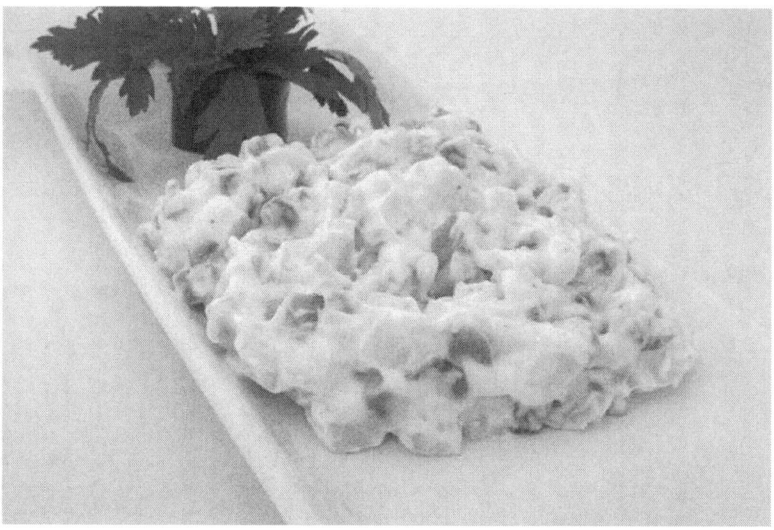

Ingredients:

1. 6 egg yolks.
2. 2 cup olive oil.

3. 2 tbsp vinegar.
4. 2 tbsp mustard wholegrain.
5. Salt and pepper to taste.

Instruction:

1. Pour egg yolk in a bowl. Add vinegar, salt, pepper and stir until well mix.
2. Add oil, mustard grain, and some warm water into mixture and blend until thick and creamy.
3. Serve immediately and enjoy.

Keto Beef Stock

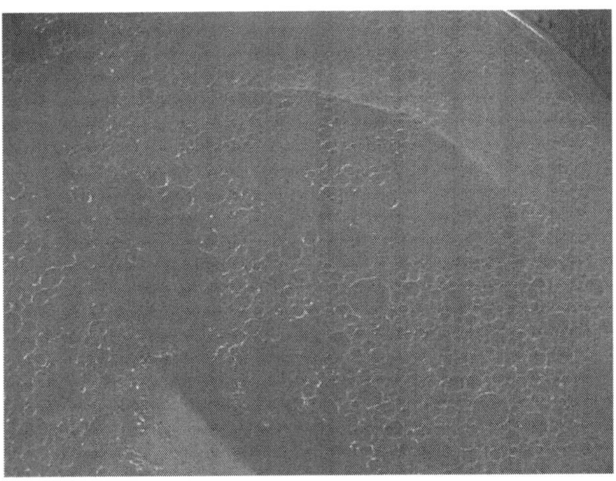

Ingredients:

1. 4 pounds beef with a shank.
2. ½ cup vegetable oil.
3. 2 large finely minced carrot.
4. 2 medium size minced onion.
5. 2 minced garlic cloves.
6. 2 tbsp minced parsley.
7. Salt and ground pepper to taste.

Instruction:

1. Season beef with salt and pepper. Add water and cook until nearly done.
2. Heat oil in a pan. Pour cooked beef with broth and stir.
3. Add onion, garlic, parsley, carrot. Stir and allow to cook over medium heat.
4. Reduce heat and add little more water, salt, pepper, stir and simmer until done.
5. Serve immediately and enjoy.

Keto Classic Caesar Dressing

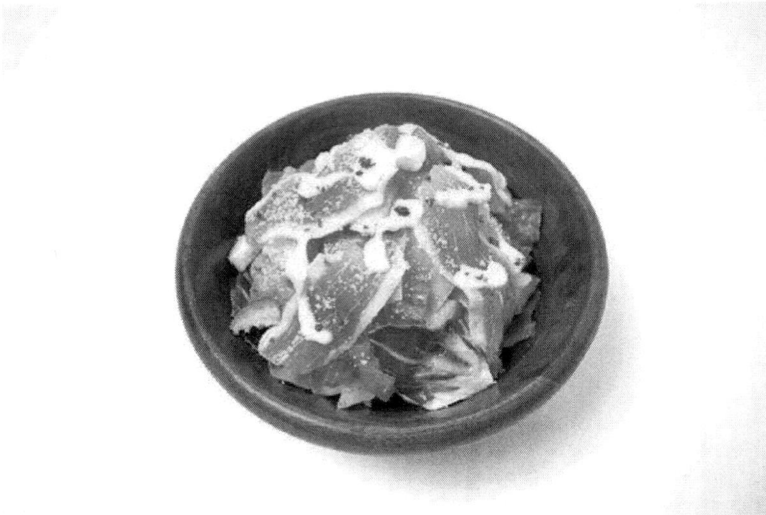

Ingredients:

1. 1 cup parmesan cheese.
2. 1 pounds shredded bacon.
3. 3 egg yolks.
4. 1 large shredded sourdough bread.
5. 1 tbsp mustard.
6. ½ cup olive oil.
7. 1 tbsp vinegar.
8. ½ cup shredded anchovies.
9. 1 large well minced lettuce head.
10. 2 garlic minced garlic cloves.
11. Salt and ground black pepper to taste.

Instruction:

1. Preheat oven to 190^{oc}.
2. Put the egg yolk in a food processor to make Caesar dressing. Add vinegar, garlic, mustard, anchovy, oil, and blend. Add salt, pepper, and process until smooth. Pour into a container, cover and refrigerate.
3. Place bread on a tray, coat bread with oil and sprinkle salt and pepper over bread. Bake for 10 minutes until golden and set aside.
4. Heat oil in a pan and add bacon. Stir-cook for 5 minutes until golden then set aside to drain.
5. Place lettuce in a bowl. Add cheese, season with little salt and pepper and toss. Add Caesar dressing and bacon and toss until well combined.
6. Serve immediately and enjoy.

Chicken Stock with Herb

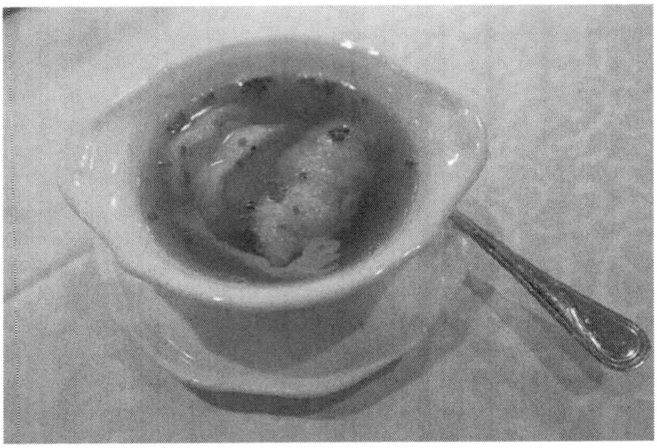

Ingredients:

1. 2 pounds cut fresh chicken meat.
2. 2 tbsp minced basil.
3. 2 tbsp minced celery.
4. 2 tbsp minced thyme.
5. 1 tbsp minced rosemary.
6. 2 large chopped carrots.
7. 4 tbsp well minced scallion.
8. 1 minced onion.
9. 2 minced garlic cloves.
10. Salt and ground pepper as desired to taste.

Instruction:

1. Season chicken meat with salt and pepper. Add other spice and cook with plenty water for broth. Drain and reserve broth aside.
2. Pour broth into the pot. Add basil, celery, scallion, garlic, onion; cover and cook over medium heat.
3. Reduce heat add cooked chicken, carrot, rosemary, thyme, salt, pepper; cover and simmer for 40 minutes. Add more water if necessary.
4. Serve immediately and enjoy.

If you have enjoyed this book, can you please take a minute and write an honest review. This kind gesture of yours will help get this book out to many other people.

1st Edition

Michael Crow

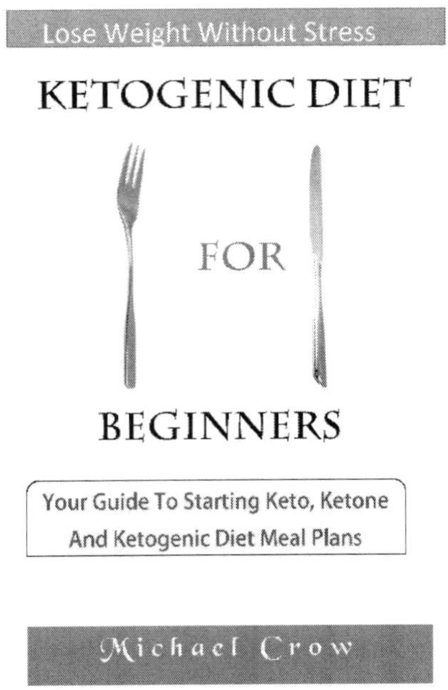

<u>Ketogenic Diet For Beginners</u>

Glossary

C

D

M

N

O

P

27301880R00232

Printed in Great Britain
by Amazon